D1557816

THERAPIST

THERAPIST

ELLEN ◇ PLASIL

ST. MARTIN'S / MAREK
NEW YORK

Design by Mina Greenstein

Library of Congress Cataloging in Publication Data

Plasil, Ellen.
   Therapist.

      1. Plasil, Ellen. 2. Psychotherapy patients—New York
(State)—Biography. 3. Psychotherapist and patient.
4. Psychotherapy patients—Abuse of. 5. Leonard, Lonnie.
6. Psychotherapists—Sexual behavior. 7. Psychotherapy
patients—Sexual behavior. I. Title.
RC464.P54A84   1985   364.1'68   85-1877
ISBN 0-312-79912-8

First Edition

10 9 8 7 6 5 4 3 2 1

TO GREG,
whose existence is testimony to Life's goodness

Contents

ACKNOWLEDGMENTS

I gratefully acknowledge my debt to Anne Kaplan for her explanations of all the legal terms, proceedings, and documents, and her interpretation of their relative importance. I am also very grateful to Maria Rivera, who helped me acquire all the necessary documents and transcripts.

Deepest appreciation is extended to my husband. Not only did he never complain about the innumerable nights spent alone while I kept company with my typewriter, he offered constant encouragement, invaluable editorial advice, and served as proofreader for each rewritten copy. Above all, he was always there when the pain of living through these events again got to be too much.

Finally, my thanks to Jack Moore, Ph.D., for telling me that I could write this story myself. Had I not valued his ideas and opinions, I might never have tried.

ON THE USE OF QUOTATION MARKS AND DATES

There are some words that have been spoken to me during the course of my life that I will never forget—no matter how hard I may sometimes try. (The reader will probably recognize which words and phrases those are without any difficulty.) They are stored in memory exactly as they were delivered at their moment of origin. The quotation marks around *those* words represent a verbatim conveyance.

But most conversations in this book, as in life, were remembered by their essence. It was the meaning of the communication that was retained, not the precise sentences that were used to declare it. It is, therefore, only the meaning that can be relayed to the reader. I have reconstructed those conversations as close to verbatim as is possible, but human memory being what it is, I cannot claim verbatim accuracy of all the dialogue. I do, however, claim complete accuracy of the meaning of the speaker's message as I heard it and recall it. So, except for those phrases that are burnt into memory forever, and except where I have quoted from a written record, the quotation marks serve to represent my recollection of the dialogues and not the exact words that were used.

License was also taken in the identification of some therapy sessions in that the date given for a particular therapy session may sometimes represent more than that one session. As my therapy occurred in real life, some similar sessions ran so close together in time and in content, that distinguishing one from another was either not necessary or possible. In those cases, I have merged two or more such sessions into one, but only when I was certain of the date of at least one of those sessions, the close time proximity between two or more of them, and a similar, if not identical, subject matter. Such liberty had no substantive effect on the story.

ON THE ISSUE OF PRIVACY

All of the major characters in this story are referred to by their real names. It was necessary, however, to use fictitious names for some of the minor characters. The names that are *not* real are italicized when they first appear in the text and are italicized in their first usage only.

THERAPIST

"The motive and purpose of my writing
is *the projection of an ideal man.*"

AYN RAND, *The Goal of My Writing*

1

THE◇PROBATION

December 5, 1972

"You're scum," he muttered slowly with quiet venom. "You're real scum."

His eyes, already filled with rage, bulged in their sockets as he held me hard in his stare. He paused, carefully considering his next words while filling the room with a deathly silence that forewarned what was yet to come.

"I'm thinking about throwing you out." He said it seriously, as if there were a puzzle for him to solve before reaching his conclusion. He was not merely trying to frighten me. "While I think about what to do, you're going to stay right where you are and listen to everything I have to say to you. *That* is the first punishment for what you've done."

Before he could continue his judgment and sentence, I moved from the chair on which I was seated across from him and knelt on the floor. My hands were clasped in front of me as I began to beg for what seemed to be my life.

"Please don't throw me out," I whispered in desperation. "I'm begging you." I had begun to cry softly, so I looked at the floor to hide my eyes—and to escape his. "I'm sorry. Really

---

1

sorry. I'll do anything to make it up to you, but *please*, please don't throw me out."

"If I don't throw you out, your begging and tears won't be the reason for it."

Then he looked at me as if he finally knew what he wanted to say. He took a deliberate pause. Then he spoke.

"You're not even half the woman I thought you were—and I didn't think you were much to start with."

I waited for him to speak the words I had dreaded, but when only silence followed, I asked him for the decision that I knew was implied. "Does this mean that you're throwing me out?" My eyes still hugged the floor as I spoke.

"I'm still thinking about it," he answered curtly.

It had been a mistake for me to speak. I should have known better by now. So I waited quietly for him to recommence his judgment on me. After all, if there was even a glimmer of hope that he might pardon me, I did not want my behavior during this hour to be the last straw that convinced him otherwise.

"You know," he continued, "you violated my first rule. You didn't tell me everything that was going on inside your head. You didn't tell me about the guilt, the doubts, or this turmoil you say you were experiencing. And all of this over what? A little sex?"

I was stunned. After all the times I had tried to discuss my reactions and feelings with him, I could not believe what I was hearing now. But I did not dare open my mouth. Nor did I dare challenge his measurement of "a *little* sex."

"I really overestimated you as a woman. Bad judgment on my part." The latter statement was said more to himself than to me. "Your future is over," he warned, "unless I agree to continue seeing you. You know that, don't you?"

"I know," I replied in a whisper. I really believed it.

"I had been sensing for some time now that you were progressing slowly. You seemed—strange. This was it, wasn't it? You just couldn't handle it. You couldn't handle the closeness and the physical contact.

"Do you know how low you are?" he asked me. He was no longer talking to himself; he wanted me to answer.

"Yes, sir, I do."

"I don't think you really do. You're scum." Then he asked, "Do you think you're scum?"

"Yes, sir, I do." Now I was crying hard.

Then, as if a lightbulb had gone off in his head, he abruptly announced his decision. "I'll let you stay," he announced. "As punishment to me, I'll let you stay. Seeing your face on a regular basis will be the price I will have to pay for having misjudged you better than you really are.

"I had thought you were more mature—more feminine. I'll pay for that mistake by subjecting myself to your presence every other week." He mulled over his words for a moment and then added, "Yes, that's fair."

He continued. "This punishment for me will be a *probation* for you. Your probation will last one year, perhaps longer.

"Probation means that you will do exactly what I tell you to do. You will do it when and how I want it done. You will tell me everything that is going on in your life and in your head. You will push yourself to improve, or you're out. You will progress faster than anyone else, or you're out. You will obey me, or you're out. And if you so much as look like you're relaxing in here, you're out."

When he stopped listing the terms and conditions of my probation, I looked up from the floor. My eyes hooked on his. He locked my glance and asked deliberately, "Is that clear?"

"Yes, sir."

"And besides your probation, there will be a second punishment."

"Yes?"

"I will never touch you again, nor allow you to touch me. Not for the rest of my life."

I did not respond, but our eyes remained fixed on each other for what seemed to be a very long time.

Even though there was still time left, he informed me that I should leave, sarcastically adding, ". . . unless you want to complain about not getting your money's worth."

I said nothing and rose from the floor. I needed tissues for my eyes and nose, but I did not help myself to those on his desk. I didn't deserve them.

I went directly home after that session with my psychiatrist and contemplated methods of suicide.

2

NEW ◇ BEGINNINGS

January 6, 1972

The day for which I had waited so long had finally arrived. I embarked on my day's venture early in the morning, arriving at the Yonkers train station with more than a half hour to spare. I used the time to review the events of the last seven months that had brought me to this moment.

A year and a half after my marriage, six months after my twentieth birthday, and several months before the birth of my son, nagging anxiety and periodic episodes of depression began approaching a level of severity and a degree of frequency I had known from a different time in my life—a time I never wanted repeated. It seemed that the few brief years I had just had of contentment, even happiness, were slipping away. And it was maddening.

It was not so much the painful anxiety and depression which I found myself increasingly reexperiencing that concerned me as it was the awareness that happiness was, once again, eluding me. Why had the therapy undergone in my teens not effected a permanent result? Why could I not hold on to that feeling of well-being and satisfaction that others seemed to take for granted? The only thing that seemed not to fade during those years was the fierce conviction that happiness could be mine and that therapy was the means to that goal.

Psychotherapy carried with it no stigma for me. It had always been the normal course of action for those in my life who suffered their own kind of anguish. There was no shame in anguish, I thought, only in the refusal to do something about it.

I wanted more than the mere semblance of happiness and success. I always had. I wanted to feel connected and in touch with my feelings. I wanted to experience a sense of continuity between my past and my present. I wanted to feel pleasure as deeply as I felt pain, but an absence of pain was as close as I could come lately to feeling pleasure. I wanted more. I wanted to be happy to be alive—and I was not.

There was a desperation to these desires. It came not only from a need to rid myself of the pain, but from a moral code that dictated that one should never accept less for one's life than what one believed was possible. The pain I felt and the code I accepted, coupled with the naïveté and idealism of my youth, sent me looking for new answers. I thought, I hoped, that the answer would be found in a new therapy.

I learned about Objectivist Psychology through the writings of Allan Blumenthal, M.D., and Nathaniel Branden. Both contributed articles to the monthly newsletter devoted to Ayn Rand's philosophy of *Objectivism*, to which my father held a subscription. My introduction to Objectivism was made by my father during my middle teens and my exposure was limited to the books and articles with which my father provided me. This was augmented only by dinnertime dialogues with my father. By my late teens, however, I was introduced—quite by accident—to a whole social structure revolving around Objectivism and, eventually, my entire support system of friends and acquaintances came to be composed of men and women who embraced the same ideology as I. At least, so they said and so I believed.

Having made the decision to reenter therapy, my natural choice for a therapist was Dr. Blumenthal. The fact that he practiced in New York City and I lived in the Midwest didn't daunt me. I would simply move my husband, baby, and myself out East.

But when I telephoned Dr. Blumenthal to discuss my intentions, my hopes were quickly dashed.

"My waiting list for new patients is three years long," he politely informed me.

"Three years?" I asked, hoping I had heard him wrong. "I can't wait three years." I paused a moment to search for options. "Can you recommend anyone else?" I asked.

"Yes," he replied, "there is a doctor I can recommend. Actually, he is the *only* psychiatrist I would recommend."

I should have felt renewed encouragement. I may not have been getting an appointment with the eminent Dr. Allan Blumenthal, but I was getting the next best thing: the name of a therapist whom Dr. Blumenthal could highly recommend. But all I felt was disappointment. As he spoke, I scribbled the name he gave me on a piece of scrap paper and halfheartedly promised to consider the idea.

In the weeks that followed, my situation did not improve. My marriage, in which I had been unhappy from the beginning, was causing increased discontentment. I felt trapped in the relationship, and those feelings were exacerbated by my new baby's demands.

My frustration was only heightened by my friends' exodus to New York. They, too, were familiar with Dr. Blumenthal's work and saw the answer to their happiness in his office. Young and single, they were free to move without any consideration of family obligations and without any advance planning. But whereas their departures had underscored my loneliness, their visits home or by phone accentuated my impatience for a better and happier life. They had left Chicago for therapy with Dr. Blumenthal, but learning of his three-year waiting list upon their arrival, most opted to seek therapy from the man whom

Dr. Blumenthal was recommending. They were now spreading the word.

Their therapist, they believed, would do nothing short of revolutionizing psychotherapy. They were filled with enthusiasm and raved endlessly about their new doctor. Superlatives ranged from "brilliant" to "genius," from "innovative" to "renegade." They claimed to be happier than ever and growing more so every day. They each considered it their greatest good fortune that Dr. Blumenthal's waiting list had been so long.

I listened eagerly to the hours of conversation that revolved around the therapist in New York City. I hung on every word as my friends seemed to share, more with one another than with the outsiders still living in Chicago, the prize they had found out East.

I cannot count the times I heard: "He has changed my life." I do know that somewhere amid all the accolades, I became convinced that he would change my life, too. I was ready to be saved.

I called the name I had scribbled on that small piece of paper. He, too, informed me of a waiting list, but six months was far more tolerable than three years had been. The countdown, however, would not commence until my arrival in New York.

Not wanting to waste any more of my life than was necessary, we were packed and relocated within weeks. I phoned my new therapist to announce my arrival, and the six-month countdown was underway.

Those six months were filled with more stories and examples of his work. My friends continued not only to praise the therapy and the man, but began to point out to me, with a great lack of sensitivity and tact, those personality traits in me that definitely required the assistance of someone like their psychiatrist. In the tone of the message was the implication that they had become better—not only better than they had been when they started therapy, but better than—superior to—those who had not yet started, or those who had started with a different doctor. This attitude did not repel me. It merely made me more impatient to become one of them.

During these months, I saw their airs of superiority not for what they were, but as a sign of their improving self-confidence and self-esteem. I did not consider their constant praise of their therapist as a sign of unnatural allegiance or loyalty, but as a testament to his fine work and skill. My friends were well on their way to a better life, and I could only count the days to my new beginning. How appropriate, I tried to console myself, that my six months would be up with the turning of the new year. A new year, a new beginning, a new life.

As I boarded the train on that early day in January and prepared to make the last leg of this journey to my new therapist, I was filled with enormous anticipation, excitement, and dreams of a happiness I was yet to know. As the train made its way from Yonkers to Manhattan, my impatience for this ride to end mounted. Those forty minutes seemed interminable. Only the written train schedule in my hand assured me that there was, indeed, a destination point for this train.

Yes, today was a great day. Today would change my life forever. Today, I would finally meet him: Lonnie Franklin Leonard, M.D.

3

RECOLLECTIONS

During the train ride, I thought of what my first session would bring. My new therapist would probably ask me first, as the psychiatrists before him had, about my childhood and family background. So I reviewed the chronology of my past, drifting in and out of daydreams that made these recollections almost come to life.

The thread of my life did not begin until I was nine years old. Not that I could remember, anyway. My memories of the years before were often sketchy, disconnected, and incomplete. There was certainly nothing solid enough to give me a sense of where I had come from, or of any continuity.

Whereas so much of my past could not be remembered, there were fleeting images, sounds, and scenes which could not be forgotten. I held very strong images of my mother from those years. I could still see the cold fire in her eyes, the frenzied flurry of her arms, and the shaking of her body fat as she went storming through our apartment. And now, on the train, I could hear Mommy screaming, children crying, and doors slamming, but as in most of my visual recollections, I could not recall the specific instances from which these memories had been taken.

Of my father during those early years, I had only one general memory: his silent witness to my mother's abuse. And it was with the recollection of this image on the train that memories of who *I* had been during those years and after were triggered. Now I was remembering how my mother's treatment of me and how my father's passivity had enraged me as a child, and that my anger had been freely and frequently expressed. Perhaps, it occurred to me now, that was why it had always been so easy for me in later years to speak out when I witnessed other examples of people's cruelty or irrationality. I had begun to fight back at a very early age, stamping that personality trait into the mold of who I was and how I saw myself. But I had been more than a fighter. More than that had been necessary to survive.

I would not be able to tell my new therapist how young I had been when I first began to hear from adults that I was *too* serious, *too* pensive, *too* sensitive. I would, however, be able to tell him that, whatever the *too* was meant to criticize, the adjectives had been quite accurate. Even as I sat riding on this train into the city, the strongest memory I had of myself in early childhood was that of a little girl always struggling to understand the confusion around her. Making sense out of a world that seemed crazy had occupied much of my time. Trying to understand why Mommy thought me to be crazy had occupied much of the rest of it.

"I don't think I'm crazy," I told her.

"The first sign of insanity, Ellen, is when you think that you're okay and that the rest of the world is crazy," she answered.

It was not, however, these explicit questions on my sanity that caused me to truly doubt the functioning of my mental faculties. Those remarks had been delivered with the ambiguous tone of half seriousness, half jest. I never knew if she had or had not meant to communicate as truth the implied conclusion with which I had been left. What caused the most concern and confusion for me was my mother's authoritative psychoanalysis of me during our disagreements. While I needed to understand *the facts* of a situation, my mother remained focused on *my psychology*.

"What you're really angry at," she would add after our screaming at each other had run its course, "is yourself." With an air of certainty that told me she knew my motives better than I might ever hope to, she pronounced her analysis the way a judge might a verdict. "You're just mad that you got caught," she might have decided.

"Got caught at what?" I would scream back. "What did I do? Why are you mad at me?"

"If you were honest with yourself, you'd know," she would answer.

But I didn't know. And most of the time I was left with a sense that there were bad things hidden inside of me that I could not see, but to which my mother apparently had a pipeline. She knew my *real* motives. I knew only my rage and confusion.

These kinds of instances were compounded by the ones that occurred in the calm of everyday living. Perhaps it was when I was preparing to leave the house for a visit with a friend whom she had said I could see, or when I approached her to clarify the particulars of a promise she had made for something she was to buy for me. Whatever the specific occasion was, it was often concluded with her denials that such permission or promises had been given.

"But you said so, Mommy," I would argue. And I would tell her when she had said it and what her words had been.

"You only think I said it, Ellen," she would answer. "You only *think* you know what I said. You can't ever really know it. And you are thinking wrong."

That I could not make her address the issues for which I needed explanations, infuriated me. That she turned our discussions and arguments against my psychology, frustrated me. That she so often denied having said what I so clearly remembered her saying, angered me. And that she taught me that my perceptions could never be certain, but that only my misperceptions of reality could be, scared me. Slowly I came to doubt my own mental processes, the words I felt so certain I had heard and the actions I could have sworn were taken. But while I grew to question my sanity, I never let go of the outrage provoked by her mistreatment of me.

When I was unable to resolve the puzzle of a particular incident, or unable to discern what was true from what she wanted me to believe was true, I would handle the pain of my frustration, anger, and confusion in one of two ways. The first was to enter into a silent dialogue with my many stuffed animals, reasoning out the rights and wrongs of the problem at hand with them. There were fourteen of them in all. We gathered every night in my bed, after the lights in the rest of the apartment had gone out, and there we exchanged our ideas on the happenings of the day. Just as importantly, we showed our love for one another.

Each animal represented, through its own unique personality, a particular perspective on any given problem. Once I had presented the issue to the group of animals, each would come forward with his analysis. Lassie, my stuffed collie, always saw things from the perspective of fairness.

"Do you think I should have been hit for that?" I would ask the group.

"No," Lassie would answer, "it's not fair to hit children if they didn't do anything wrong."

Peter, my stuffed blue rabbit, on the other hand, looked out for the other side.

"She is your mother," Peter often reminded me. "Even if you don't know what you did wrong, maybe your mother does."

Cocoa, my brown bear, was a timid soul, and dreaded any sort of physical violence, especially against children.

"It doesn't matter if she did do anything wrong," Cocoa would argue with Peter. "It's never right to hit children."

And so these discussions would go, often until late into the night. I had suffered from insomnia since before I can remember and those restless nights were not wasted. My stuffed animals were my friends and allies inside those apartment walls, and the dialogues I had with them inside my head were my way of finding comfort and reason in a world where they were absent.

My alternate method of dealing with any particular day's trauma was to write down my own judgment about the matter in the spiral notebook that served as my diary, followed by promises never to behave that way when I grew up.

—I will never chase my children around the house.
—I will never corner my children while swinging my arms at them.
—I will never hit my children without telling them why.
—I will never hate my children.
—I will never have a little girl because little girls are always sad.

And when Mommy decided that I was too old to have stuffed animals anymore, I wrote in my spiral notebook:

—I will never throw away my children's toys.

Whereas some of my memories were hazy and vague, I could not recall ever not feeling that I had been singled out by my mother as her favorite target for cruelty. It was not the physical *punishments* which I seemed to receive more than my brother and sister that told me of this difference between them and me. It was even more than her hostile words or confusing arguments. It was, rather, the way in which she looked at me that demonstrated her true feelings toward me. Yet, this was the most difficult element for me, as a child, to identify and understand. I could *feel* the message in my mother's attitude, but to name it for what it felt like would have been too incredible for belief—and too painful. Five years from now, it would be my mother who would finally put into words what I had felt to be the case for so long. But now my mind wandered to one of those instances in which it had been her eyes and tone of voice that had said as much, if not more, than her words.

I recalled the summer of my eighth year, when I had just returned home from my first summer at overnight camp. I had come home feeling so proud and excited, for the day before I had taken first place in my division of the camp's horse show. Daddy had introduced me to riding and I was the only family member to share his passion for the sport. I had not slept a wink during the night's train ride back to the city, as my anxiousness to see Daddy's face when he saw my blue ribbon kept me from relaxing.

I checked to see that the ribbon was securely fastened to the center of my blouse, where it had been since I boarded the train the night before, and disembarked hoping it would be the first thing Daddy would see when he greeted me. His response was nothing less than I had hoped for, and we spoke of little else during the car ride back home than stories of the competition the day before.

My mother awaited my arrival in the kitchen, where she was preparing brunch. I was still beaming and reeling from my news. I threw my arms around her and shared my achievement with her. But within moments, and for reasons I could not understand, she was growing angry. Harsh words began to fly and voices began to rise. But it was my mother who had the last word.

"This family was so much happier when you weren't here," she whispered to me.

As usual, it was not only her sharp words that stabbed at my heart. It was the coldness in her voice, the conviction in her tone, and the hatred in her eyes that disarmed me the most. And it was her manner, not her words, that brought a trembling to my body now, as I relived that incident.

As I grew older, the words she spoke, the tone she used, changed to fit my increasing level of understanding and maturity. But the message remained the same. I was an adult with a child of my own, the day she spoke to me of her will and my inheritance. While she stood primping in front of her bedroom mirror, she casually remarked that the will had been drawn, and without moving her eyes from the mirror and without changing the nonchalance in her voice, she continued to explain her reason for mentioning the subject.

"I want you to know that I showed my diamonds to your sister and let her select what she liked. You'll get what she didn't choose."

To have shown my pain, to have questioned her tact, or to have revealed the deep insult I felt, might have been interpreted as dissatisfaction with the inheritance itself. And I could not risk having this issue turned against me with accusations reminiscent of the past, as I was already too close to tears.

"What you're really angry at, Ellen, is the value of your inheritance," I could almost hear her saying. "It's not me you're angry with; you're jealous of your sister."

I did not want to have to defend my hurt feelings or my anger at her for wanting to hurt me. I did not want to listen to her analysis of my motives and pain. So I said nothing.

My father's contribution to the confusion and rage I experienced during those earlier years took the form of reinforcing silence, as well as blind obedience to his wife's demands. One of the clearest memories I held was not that of one specific instance, but of a series of identical ones, all blended into one recollection. During numerous dinner hours, Mommy, for no known or spoken reason, would rise from her place at the dinner table, and storm out of the room in silence. After her bedroom door had been heard to slam shut and lock, my father would rise in turn and chase after her. Daddy would knock on the locked door, begging for admission. Then his apologies could be heard to follow his pleas.

"I'm sorry, Honey," he would call to Mommy from the other side of the door. "Whatever it is I did, I'm really sorry."

I would turn to my sister for a sign that someone understood what was happening. "What did he do?" I would ask her. But her silence told me that she was as baffled and disturbed by the incident as I.

Daddy was often sorry for unknown sins, but by the time I was ten or eleven, I stopped trying to understand what his crime had been for which he had felt so compelled to apologize. Instead, I grew to resent the weakness that permitted Daddy to be so manipulated by Mommy.

His subservience to her whims, his obedience to her demands, were all the more confusing to me because of the contradiction between his actions and his words. It was Daddy who had been my first teacher of philosophy, ethics, and morality. Long before I was old enough to comprehend the content of such lectures, and well into the years when I could, Daddy spent endless hours teaching me the conceptual tools for survival.

A man must always think for himself, he professed. A man cannot be influenced or swayed by the opinions of another. He must form independent judgments of the events around him and stand by those judgments when called upon to do so; the first, he said, paves the road to one's pride, the second to integrity.

Logic and reason, he taught me, were the tools to understanding the world around me. A clear line existed between *right* and *wrong*, *morality* and *immorality*, and those tools would help me to see the difference as I matured.

He discussed politics, systems of government, and various philosophers, always trying to lead me to an understanding of each and a judgment on all. And when I was too small to comprehend these bigger issues, he still managed to find many examples to his lessons that fit the universe of a small child. When it rained, for example, and I refused to wear my rubber boots "because none of the other kids had to wear them," he found an opening for a demonstration.

"We don't do what other people do, Ellen," he reminded me. "We do what is right." He outlined the reasoning behind wearing rubber boots, pointing out that the rain would make my feet wet if I didn't. Then, after reminding me that wet feet can lead to colds, he would ask, "Don't you want to do what makes sense?" I wore my boots.

So when my father pandered to my mother, catered to her whims, and ignored her abuses of her children, I was confused by this man of independent judgment and integrity. And when he followed her orders to hit me, I was even more so.

"Go in there and hit her," Mommy greeted Daddy at the door one evening.

I could hear his footsteps as he approached the door to my bedroom. I heard him pose no questions or requests for an explanation to my mother. I heard only his silence and the nearing of his steps.

"Daddy," I begged as he opened the door, "she's already hit me. Do I have to get hit again?" I began to cry.

He moved toward my bed and beckoned me to his lap. "Daddy, I don't even know what I did. Can't you just ask her what I'm being punished for?"

My words did not delay nor sway him from performing the task he had been sent to do. And when I questioned him about the *rightness* of hitting a child for no known reason, about the *rightness* of getting hit twice for the same mysterious sin, about the *rightness* of the action he was about to undertake without any understanding of its purpose, he had only one response: "Your mother told me to do it." Soon after, I would receive his lecture on the nature of Nazi Germany and the consequences of an immoral code which preached the virtue of following orders. My confusion worsened.

There was only once that I could recall when Daddy's spankings had been accompanied by an anger that I had previously associated solely with my mother. It was at a time in my early adolescence when, once again, he had been ordered to hit me. While I prepared for him to come home from the office and braced myself for the punishment that I knew would come, I promised myself that this time I would not cry. I resolved not to give them the satisfaction of watching me suffer again for a crime that had not been made clear to me.

18

Daddy walked to my room after receiving his orders from Mommy at the front door, and ordered me to his lap. Without an argument, I walked to where he was seated on my bed and waited for him to pull me over his lap. Then he spanked me hard, maybe eight times, while I winced and bit my lower lip. But I did not cry.

After a few seconds of no sounds from me, Daddy spoke angrily.

"What's the matter? Wasn't it hard enough for you? You want more?"

I said nothing in reply to his questions. I was still pinned across his lap and he began to spank me again, harder and longer than the first time. As his hand developed a certain rhythm as it fell to my buttocks, I kept myself from crying out by repeating in my head *I will not cry, I will not cry*, in a sing-song pattern marked to the beat of his hand.

This time when he had finished and I was still not crying, he became infuriated. His face grew red and his body began to shake. Then he screamed, "I'll hit you till you cry! And you *will* cry!"

Once again, I tried to find the beat of his hand, to concentrate on the rhythm rather than on the pain, but I could not find the tempo. I struggled to find something else to focus on, but all I could feel was the anger in his legs that shook beneath me and the contact of his hand that was over me. Finally, I cried.

I did not know why it had been so important to him to break my will. I did not know why my determination made him so furious. I only knew that I had never hated him more than I did that evening. And I never forgot it, either.

But if I was ostracized by my mother and baffled by my father, I was also comforted by my father's obvious love for me. If I was my mother's target for abuse, I was also my father's object of affection. It had been the love and attention that I had received from Daddy that kept me glued to my chair throughout all of his lectures on *right* and *wrong, justice* and *mercy, capitalism* and *communism,* and *individualism* and *collectivism.* I alone had been singled out for these pearls of wisdom from my father, and I relished every moment of it. I thought back to those times we had spent alone and recollected the patience he seemed to take in guiding my life. He always seemed to have the time for intellectual discussion or political dialogue; he had time for me. His company was usually a bastion of sanity and calm for me, reassuring me that I was indeed loved.

Even this solace of my father's love, however, did not go without confusion. As I recalled on my ride into New York, it was sometime during my ninth year when I was awakened by my father's arms lifting me out of my bed. The apartment was dark and still, and I was disturbed by my father's bizarre behavior at that late hour.

"Where are we going, Daddy?" I whispered to him as we passed my sister's bed.

"Shhh," was his only reply.

When we had reached the vacant maid's room adjacent to the bedroom I shared with my sister, Daddy placed me on the bed and returned to the door through which we had just come. I watched as he closed the door and moved to join me on the bed. Then he began to kiss me in a funny way, in a way he had never done before. My face was getting wet from his mouth and, for some reason that I could not recall now, I had been unable to wipe my face dry as his kisses continued. I could vaguely remember his tongue at my mouth, but could not decide if that had been the source of the choking sensation I so vividly recalled.

During the train ride, I wanted so much to remember more of that night, but I felt grateful for any memory of this event at all. That night had been totally forgotten by the next morning, and was not to return to me until several years later. But even with its return to consciousness, that night still held many mysteries. I could not recall the remainder of the night. I could not even recall how I had gotten back to my own bed.

The only other memory I had of that night of which I felt sure, was of the words my father spoke to me at some point during the encounter.

"We don't ever want to tell anyone about this, Ellen. They might not understand. Your brother and sister might think that you're more special than they are and that would hurt them very much."

I did not know if these words had been spoken at the beginning or at the end of our time in that room. I could not be sure for how long he had communicated this implied order to keep silent. I was only positive about the message and of some of the words he had spoken to communicate it.

My father had rarely touched me before that night in the maid's room. He was not a demonstrative man, and any kind of parental stroking or hugging seemed to be difficult for him. But, it seemed to me now in hindsight, that he had touched me even less after that night than he had before. And, for some strange reason, even given what had occurred, I had missed that from him. He had been my primary source of comfort and love, and now I saw that our bond had been strained.

It was the recollection of my eleventh year that evoked the most vivid memories of my growing unhappiness. This was the year in which my deepening depression and growing confusion peaked. I felt abandoned by my mother and betrayed by my father. Feeling alone, bewildered, and doomed, I looked for an alternative to the life I was leading.

As I saw it then, I had three options; my mother had frequently posed the first two. I could remain the person I was— serious, pensive, depressed, argumentative—and be left alienated and friendless, at best, or deemed *different* and crazy, at worst; or, I could make a concerted effort to become normal, like her. Before I had discovered the third option, I had spent considerable time deciding whether or not I should like to be like Mommy. I had watched her for years, and, trying not to be affected by her particularly hostile treatment of me, deliberated that option carefully.

I watched as she shrieked at her family for reasons they rarely could comprehend. I watched as she ate her way through the days, growing progressively more obese each year. I watched as she ran through the apartment, either in silent rage or in bellowing anger. And I watched as she moved with schizophrenic ease between blind fury with her family and saccharine kindness with her friends. These dramatic mood swings were equally evident in other areas, especially in those that concerned the relatives whom she despised. She could curse her in-laws without mercy in the privacy of her own home, sit stonily silent during the forty-minute drive to their house in the suburbs, and then emerge from the car bestowing greetings and hugs that oozed with sweetness for those she hated. My confusion worsened. So did my contempt.

I considered this option of emulating my mother. Then I moved on to my second choice. I considered remaining who I was and facing the continuing isolation, confusion, depression, and frustration. And after weighing these options that had been presented as my only ones, after contemplating existence in a world that saw Mommy as normal and me as disturbed, after considering the prospect of becoming like her or facing more of this pain in the future, I knew my life would never be happy. Thus was born my third option.

In the middle hours of an evening past my eleventh birthday, I removed a bottle of Miltown from my mother's medicine cabinet and swallowed its contents. There had not been any particular incident which had triggered this action. It was not decided nor taken on impulse, in rage, nor for revenge. Rather, decided in a state of chronic depression, it was the natural consequence of careful deliberation and the final rejection of the only two other choices I saw. Suicide was the option of my own discovery. I attempted to exercise it that night.

I was never able to remember very much about the rest of that night, and my recollection of it now, on the train, was no different than the many times I had thought about it before. I vaguely recalled being walked around in circles in the alley behind our apartment building, and with even more uncertainty, I thought I had been barefoot. At the very least, I knew my feet had been cold. My father held me up, and as I stumbled in my night clothes begging him to let me sleep, he pushed me on to more circles while urging me to stay awake. I survived that night—only to begin my rounds to psychiatrist's offices, and to try my third option twice more before my fifteenth birthday.

I would not be able to provide my new therapist with the names of all my former psychiatrists. I had been too young, it had been too long ago, and I had never stayed long enough with some of them to care about their names. Since I had been taken to these sessions against my will, I usually sat silently in the patient's chair while my psychiatrist attempted to make me speak. At the end of each hour, the doctor would dismiss me with frustration, and once I was even ordered not to return for a second visit; my silence was a waste of his time, he had said.

My parents eventually abandoned this futile drive for my involuntary psychotherapy, acknowledging that help could only be given to those who wanted it. Three years later, with only one condition attached, I wanted it. The condition: that the therapist be a woman. For some reason unknown to me at the time, I was terrified of being left alone in a room with a male adult. My condition was met, thus beginning a two-year therapeutic relationship that was to continue until my junior year of high school.

These years were better for me, not only because my therapy was helpful, but because interests outside my home began to occupy more of my time. Two factors in particular contributed to this change in focus and direction: school and Grandma.

I loved school. I enjoyed almost all of my classes and looked forward to each day with enthusiasm for the new ideas that I knew would stimulate me during those seven hours. But it was not my classes alone that accounted for my entire sense of growing satisfaction. I had few friends, but the ones I had I considered to be good ones. And I had a boyfriend—the first male with whom I was not afraid to be alone. Time spent in class, time spent after school with friends, and time spent in the evening with homework, diverted my attention to more constructive enterprises. And these made me happier than I had ever been.

Also during these years, there was a continuation and deepening of a special relationship that I shared with my paternal grandmother. Grandma was the most unpretentious, outspoken, and open woman I knew. She was often accused by my mother, who strongly disliked Grandma, of being rude and tactless. I saw her only as genuine and honest. She spoke what she thought, and she thought for herself. That made my specialness to her all the more valuable to me. And I did know how special I was to her. She made sure I knew. So it was to Grandma I went when I needed to feel loved.

I was tied to my grandma in another way, as well. It was from her that I received the only validation of my perceptions of my parents. Mommy had tried to deceive Grandma into believing that Mommy cared for her. Grandma perceived that my mother was a fake. More than that, Grandma had always suspected that there was much more going on behind our apartment walls than what met the eye.

"There's something very wrong going on in your home," she told me often. "Something is just not right."

To the little-girl fears that I carried with me into high school, which said no one but me would ever know what really went on in the privacy of our family life, Grandma's gut-level awareness that something was so amiss, was critical for me. It would, however, be many years before I felt free enough and brave enough to verify some of her suspicions. For the time being, it was enough that she was validating my experiences.

I treasured and needed those hours spent with my grandmother. I needed to see a face light up when I walked through a front door. I needed to be treated fairly, honestly, and with love. How I needed to have time spent with me, sharing old photographs, pictures she had painted long ago, and small treasures she had collected over the years. Grandma gave me what I hungered for and I adored her. The feeling was clearly reciprocated.

My therapy progressed well from the start. I found my doctor easy to talk to, but when she chose to share some of our discussions with my parents, it quickly put a limit on the extent of my disclosures.

It had only been a short time before commencing this therapy that I had recalled the sketchy facts concerning the incident with my father in the maid's room. And it was she to whom I first ever revealed the event. She diagnosed my recollection as a Freudian fantasy, typical, she said, of a pre-pubescent female. But in face of my absolute certainty that the incident had occurred as I told it, she urged me to speak to my father about it.

I waited until dinner had been finished and the family members had separated into their respective bedrooms for television viewing, reading, or homework. I called to my father from the hall outside his and my mother's bedroom, asking if I could speak to him alone. It was the most anxious moment I had ever known.

When he had joined me in the hall, I did not think to enter the living room or dining room where we could have been seated. I had to begin speaking immediately, or I feared I would not speak at all.

"Daddy, there was a night, about five or six years ago, when—"

"I know which night you're going to ask me about," he interrupted. "You were having a nightmare. Remember how you always used to have nightmares? Well, you were having one that night, so I carried you into the maid's room to keep you from waking your sister," he explained.

"I had a lot of nightmares, Daddy." I was interrupting him now. "No one ever removed me from my bed because of them."

"I always suspected that I was too affectionate with you that night," he quickly continued. "I always worried that I kissed you too much and that you might not understand it. I even told your mother about it afterward. I told her that you might have misinterpreted the affection and comfort I was trying to give you."

"Comfort?"

"Comfort. That's all I meant by it," he replied.

I struggled to find something else to say that might make him say out loud what I thought his manner was making so clear. Before I could find the right words, he spoke again.

"Does that answer what you wanted to ask me about?"

"Yes, Daddy, you've answered my question." He had. At least the important one: Was I recalling a Freudian pre-pubescent fantasy or a real situation? Whether it had only been a night of misinterpreted paternal affection, as my father claimed it to be, did not concern me at the moment. All that mattered to me—the teenager who was so used to questioning her own perceptions, her own sanity—was that I had not perceived a fantasy as reality. The incident *did* happen. I *was* carried to the maid's room by my father. I *was* kissed in such a way that made my face wet and made my father feel compelled to tell my mother about his behavior. He did something to me that night that made him know to which night I was referring before naming it. He did something to me that night that made him worry about it being "misinterpreted."

The memory, as incomplete as it was, had been fiercely strong in its imagery and feelings. But equally strong had been my therapist's words telling me that I was mistaking fantasy for reality, and my mother's words reminding me that neurotics build sandcastles in the sky while psychotics live in them. I did not live in sandcastles.

As time passed, I grew discontent with just the confirmation of my sanity. I needed to know whether that night had occurred as I remembered it. The lack of an explicit confession from my father still left me with a hint of doubt over my recollections. And that doubt was compounded by the realization that if my memory had served me correctly, my father had either repressed the details—or he had lied to me. It would take more than eighteen years after our discussion, more than eleven years after this train ride, and more than twelve years after parenting my own child, before I would be able to fully appreciate the absurdity of my father's explanation. I would think of all the times my son had needed comforting, or that I had just needed to show him my love. And I would recall how freely that comfort and affection had been given. I would think of how often I had wrapped my arms tightly around him, rocked him in my lap, kissed his gorgeous face, or even smothered him in my embraces and kisses when his cuteness was more than I could bear! And never—not even once in over twelve years of this giving of affection—did it so much as cross my mind that he could misinterpret my behavior. Never once did it occur to me to discuss the possibility of his misunderstanding my intentions with his father. And the thought of those things would have seemed beyond absurdity; they would have been laughable.

What circumstances could provoke such an idea to run through the mind of a parent? I knew the answer, and I would never, after nearly two decades of contemplating my father's words, question myself about it again.

4

THE ◇ FIRST
SESSION

The downstairs outer lobby housed the apartment building's security phone. I found LEONARD, L. F. on the code list, picked up the receiver to the push-button phone, and pressed the three-digit number beside his name.

"Hello," I heard him say.

"It's Ellen."

"I'm on the eighth floor," he explained. "Turn left off the elevator and come to the end of the hall. The door is unlocked. Just walk in and wait."

My heart was pounding so hard I thought it would come right through my chest. My palms were sweating and I was having difficulty breathing. This was it. I was almost there.

I followed his instructions and opened the door to a large, almost square room that served as vestibule, living room, and dining area. The decor was modern with a color scheme of blues and white.

A few feet ahead of me and to the left were two identical sofas facing each other and running perpendicular to a large set of windows that overlooked First Avenue between Twentieth and Twenty-third Streets. Glass tables held selected pieces of contemporary sculpted artwork, plants, and reading material.

The boundaries to this living room were marked by an oversized blue area rug and a row of low, white module units, which stored books, magazines on skiing and motorcycles, a collection of *National Geographics*, and the hi-fi from which the Henry Mancini piece was coming.

A small Scandinavian dining table lay straight ahead with four molded plastic chairs surrounding it. The dining room furniture stood on the exposed parquet floor, which also provided the walkway to the hall just beyond. The narrow hallway led, I assumed, to an office and a bathroom. Later I learned it was also the route to the bedroom.

Still standing at the front door, taking in every detail of the environment, I noticed a door to my immediate left which led to the kitchen. It was a small and very narrow room with almost no color in it save the blue of the carpet and the green of some small plants, which provided contrast to the white walls and appliances.

I closed the front door behind me and moved toward one of the sofas. Three men stood talking and laughing at the hallway entrance, apparently not noticing my presence. Suddenly, one of them turned to me and said, "Let's go."

"What?" I responded.

"Let's begin," he instructed.

I still did not understand what this man wanted. Responding to my blank stare, he replied: "I'm Lonnie Leonard."

I was stunned. I had believed him to be a patient. He looked like a patient. I was not too sure what a patient necessarily looked like, but he certainly did not look like a great doctor.

He stood maybe five feet, nine inches tall with a slim but moderately developed physique. I don't know why I had expected him to be tall and gaunt, but his shortness and unassuming presence were a surprise. I just stood there, staring at him, taking in all the contradictions to my imagined portrait of the great Dr. Leonard.

Dark hair, which had just begun to gray, topped a head with a receding hairline. His cropped Afro made his ears appear much too large for his small face. I would have guessed his age to be about forty and would not have been short by more than a year or two. His face had an impish quality about it. It reminded me of those imaginary elves I had seen in picture storybooks as a child. Had his ears only been pointed, I thought, the picture would have been more integrated. Then I caught his eyes watching me staring at him.

They were large eyes, almost circular in shape. When he raised his eyebrows, his eyes seemed to bulge some out of their sockets. To myself, and later to my more intimate friends, I would label that look "Leonard's bug eyes."

"Are you ready?" he interrupted my transfixation.

It was with that question that I perceived for the first time a slight, yet distinct southern accent. That not only added to the contradictions between prior images and reality, but made me aware of a prejudice I did not know I held. Why, I wondered, did I hold a negative correlation between intelligence and Southerners?

I moved toward the entrance of the hall where he awaited me. Upon reaching it, Dr. Leonard instructed me to remove my shoes. That's when I noticed that he was barefoot.

"My carpets," he replied to the question on my face.

I had removed my shoes and followed him down the gold carpeted hall for several feet when he turned around to face me, extended his right arm to his side, and indicated that I should precede him into the room on my left. I entered his office and awaited further instructions.

It was a small square room, also modern in decor. Floor-to-ceiling bookshelf units covered two walls, a window took up a third, and a door, chair, and file cabinet covered the fourth. A desk protruded into the room from one of the shelving units with a chair on either side of it. There was, noticeably for a psychiatrist's office, no couch.

A medical degree hung on the wall in between two of the shelves. The University of Arkansas, and his brief reference to his hometown of Little Rock, placed the drawl I had heard.

30

He told me to be seated on the straight-back chair; he took the swivel recliner behind the desk. That was when I first noticed the camera, the tape machine, and the television screens. Before another word was spoken, he put the video equipment into operation. I was now being recorded.

"Each session will be videotaped," he began. "You'll come for a session every other week, and on the *off* week, you will come to watch the recording of your previous session. If you want to, that is. You're under no obligation to see the tapes, but I do recommend it.

"As you know, I charge thirty-five dollars for each session. For viewing of tapes, I charge ten dollars. Whereas sessions are conducted in the office, tape viewings are conducted in the kitchen."

"In the kitchen?" I asked.

"Yes. There's a small Sony in there and I'll teach you how to use the tape player when you come for your first viewing. As you may have already heard—or figured out—I live as well as work here. This office is actually one of two bedrooms in the apartment. So if you should ever need to reach me, you need only to call my office number. If I am at home, I will pick up. If I am out, my machine will take your message and I'll return your call as soon as I get home." Then he added, as if to explain his system, "I have no answering service, no secretary, no receptionist, no bookkeeper. I prefer to do everything myself."

There were more rules, but these governed the process of therapy itself. It was with the recitation of these that I felt my session had actually begun.

"The patient and the therapist each have a set of responsibilities to fulfill if the patient is to benefit from the therapeutic process," he began. "Your first responsibility is to report everything you can about what is occurring in your life and in your head. Everything."

"Okay," I said to let him know that I was listening.

"This is my first rule of therapy. If I should ever discover

31

that you have failed to communicate such information to me, that will be considered grounds for dismissal."

"What?" I had heard rumors that, on occasion, Dr. Leonard had dismissed patients abruptly for some sort of bad thing, which had always gone unspecified in the rumors. Could this have been their crime? Not reporting everything to their doctor? I wondered.

"I mean this quite seriously. Therapy cannot progress unless you're doing your part. That's why this is my first rule of therapy. If the patient is not interested in getting better and working toward that goal, I don't want to waste my time. I have a waiting list of people wanting to do therapy with me, and I only want to work with those people who really want to change. That's one reason why most of my patients are young. The younger they are, the more they want and are apt to change.

"Now, do you know what monitoring is?" he asked, changing the subject and the tone of his voice.

"I think so," I answered. "It's paying attention to what you're feeling so that you know what's going on inside yourself. Right?"

"Well, it's also having an eye on your thought processes, too. It's not just a monitor of emotions," he explained. "It's a process whereby you almost stand outside yourself to see what is happening inside yourself. Are you good at monitoring?" he asked.

"I think so."

"Everyone thinks so, but most people aren't. You'll get good at it, though. Pay attention to all the signals that your subconscious feeds you. *Monitor* them. Then come in here and discuss what is coming up for you. That's your job. Any questions?"

"No."

"Well, I have one for you. What is it called when a person ignores the signals being delivered by his subconscious?"

All of a sudden I felt like I was being tested. But I knew from my readings on Objectivist Psychology and from the tone in his voice what the answer was. "Evasion?" I answered with uncertainty.

It was the one sin in which Objectivists never wanted to find themselves caught. Evasion was immoral, and even the mere suspicion of evasion usually resulted in condemnations and social excommunication. I did not have to ask Dr. Leonard what evasion would mean for future therapy.

"If you evade, needless to say, you're out. And, of course, if you lie to me, you're out. I am not a mind reader. I cannot do therapy with a patient who provides me with incomplete or false information." He was finished with his responsibilities and rules for the patient. He was ready to move on to the therapist.

"My responsibility is to assist you in identifying those emotions and thought processes that you will be experiencing. My role is to act as a teacher, explaining to you which ideas, emotions, and thought processes are correct and healthy. Remember, emotions don't come from a vacuum. They are the result of your premises. If you hold bad premises, it follows that your emotions will reflect that."

His words were familiar Objectivist jargon. I was, nevertheless, reassured by his underlying premise: It was possible for me to change; I could be happy.

"Together, we will work toward substituting your bad ideas, premises, emotions, whatever, with the healthy ones I will give you for their replacement. You understand?"

"Yes, I do."

"And finally, I am responsible for providing you with feedback on your progress. I'll let you know how you're doing."

Dr. Leonard did not state what consequences would befall him if he was negligent in *his* role.

My mood had changed since twenty minutes earlier. I was still nervous, but less from anticipation than from apprehension. I had never heard of videotaping therapy sessions before. I had never heard of rules governing the process of therapy before. I had never heard of walking barefoot into a session before. But before my anxiety could totally numb my excitement, the session took a new direction.

He began to ask probing, gentle questions about me, about my life. With an equal amount of intensity and concern, he questioned me about everything from background to present feelings, from IQ to hobbies.

"Why are you seeking therapy? Are you experiencing specific symptoms?"

I told him about my anxiety and depression, and he pressed me for more information. He wanted specific problems. He wanted details.

"The most obvious one is a sexual one," I told him. "I am unable to have orgasms."

"Did you ever consider that you might be married to the wrong man?" he asked matter-of-factly.

I did not want to admit that I had, so I let the question slide for the time being.

"I also have a phobia. A bug phobia. Spiders and roaches in particular."

"How do you react when you see them?" he inquired.

"I scream or run, whichever comes first."

He asked me about my educational background, and I told him about my private-school education and my year and a half of college. He did not ask why I had left school in my sophomore year. He continued with other questions.

"What is your family situation?" he asked next.

"Do you mean my husband and child, or my parents and siblings?"

"The latter," he answered.

Instead of explaining to him what I had reviewed on the train, I explained the present status of my relationship with my mother and father.

"Just prior to my moving here," I told him, "my mother telephoned me to say that she wanted nothing further to do with me. She said she and my father were disowning me."

"Did she say why?"

"There had been long-standing antagonism between my brother and me," I explained to him, "and we had resumed our battle during a dinner at my mother's one evening.

"I was still angry with him from our argument when he

made a move to pick up my baby, so I told him I didn't want him holding my son." I waited for Dr. Leonard's response.

"Yes?" he said. "Go on."

"That's it."

"That's what?" he asked.

"That's why my mother said they were disowning me," I answered.

"What?" He was confused. But then, he was not used to my mother.

"My mother called me on the phone after that evening—I don't remember if it was the next morning or several days later—and told me that I should not have told my brother not to hold my baby. She went on to say that, as a result, she and Daddy had decided that they could no longer associate with me.

"My husband was on the extension during the call. He had gathered from my end of the conversation what was going on, so he picked up the other phone. He pleaded with Mom to reconsider what she was doing. He told her that this was a problem to be reconciled between a brother and sister, and that he was certain it eventually would be. But she didn't listen. And he didn't understand."

"He didn't understand what?" Dr. Leonard asked.

"He didn't understand that she was just looking for an excuse."

"How did you feel while this was going on?"

"I was sort of in shock. I couldn't believe what she was doing. I also couldn't believe that my father really knew what she was up to. But I couldn't argue with her. I just let my husband do the talking, I guess because I knew from the beginning that there was no sense in trying to change her mind. I had seen my mother's extreme behavior in the past, and neither reason nor tears would have changed her mind."

Dr. Leonard looked curious. "Did your mother try to explain why she felt the need to side with one child against another?"

"She said she was doing it to defend my brother. That not taking sides would be the same thing as abandoning him."

He had listened intently as I spoke, looking down only to make notes in the folder on his desk. He had interjected occasional questions of clarification, indicating the careful attention he had been giving to my words. "But she could have taken neither side and abandoned neither child," he pondered aloud. "Did she explain why the form of her defense had to be disowning you? Did she explain why he needed defending at all?"

He looked directly at me when he spoke, releasing me from his gaze only long enough to make a notation. And it was, I suppose, this intensity with which he worked, as well as the attentiveness with which he listened that made him seem more attractive than his mere physical presence had originally. He began to emanate a certain charisma that comes with wisdom, experience, and skill. And I began, for the first time that hour, to see some of what my friends had been describing for so long.

Then, in the middle of his questioning and at the end of my description of this past phone conversation, Dr. Leonard placed his pen on his desk, leaned over on his forearms, stared directly at me, and asked with concern, "How close are the tears?"

I felt in that moment that the question itself would make me cry. I felt seen and understood. I hadn't known I was close to tears, but all of a sudden I was aware of it. He had known it before I. He had been able to see inside my soul and witness my pain. And I could tell that it mattered to him that I was hurting. It mattered to the great Dr. Leonard.

I had tried to be cool and businesslike in my descriptions, but he had seen beyond my cover. His question not only told me how perceptive he was, but his tone told me how compassionate, as well. His greatness seemed clearer to me now and my apprehension about the session disappeared. It did not occur to me that his question could have been prompted merely by the content of my last description or by the context of our meeting: a patient in pursuit of psychotherapy.

"Very," I replied.

"Yes," he said knowingly. Then he returned to the routine.

He listed a series of psychological states and asked me to evaluate myself in respect to each. Repression. Guilt. Anxiety. Hostility. Anger. Bitterness. Then again, as unexpected as it had been the first time, Dr. Leonard put down his pen, leaned across his desk, and looked at me both intently and compassionately.

"I know underneath that veneer of control and cool, there is a soft, gentle, caring, loving woman. Together we are going to work to bring her out."

With this, he was speaking to every facet of my being that had ever wanted to be seen by other people. Of course I am warm and loving inside; of course I am gentle and caring, I thought. But how did he see that? How wonderful he must be, indeed, to see those things that lay so deep inside me being protected from outside dangers. How insightful he must be to see that part of me that I experience as my core. Again, he had seen my soul. This time he saw its beauty, just as he had seen its pain.

Before the hour ended, Dr. Leonard gave me a homework assignment. Eighty-seven incomplete sentences filled two typewritten pages. I was to complete the sentences and hand them in before or at my next session. I knew I would do my assignment before the day's end. After all, I wanted to progress quickly. I wanted to get down to work. And I wanted to impress my doctor.

The top of the page gave the instructions:

Some incomplete sentences are listed below. Read each one and make it into a complete sentence by writing out the first thing that comes into your mind. Work as rapidly as you can. If you cannot complete an item, circle its number and return to it later. If necessary, use the back of the sheet to complete sentences, and correctly number any sentence completed there.

I dated the page January 6th, and began.

Many of the sentences carried little significance for me, but I finished them with earnestness nonetheless.

SENTENCE 1. I like . . . *to sing.*
SENTENCE 2. When I am happy I . . . *sing.*

Some sentences were a reflection of my present state of mind. For example, my optimism as a result of commencing therapy that day with Dr. Leonard is seen in:

SENTENCE 79. I think that the best years are . . . *ahead.*

Similarly, others told of my purpose and reason for pursuing therapy and, at the same time, of my life's focus during this period.

SENTENCE 3. I want to know . . . *why I am not always happy.*
SENTENCE 14. I want most . . . *to be happy—really happy.*
SENTENCE 45. I could be perfectly happy . . . *if I were perfectly happy.*
SENTENCE 49. What I want most in the world is . . . *to be happy.*

Two of the sentences, however, were extremely significant. They did not seem so at the time, but later they would be seen as such in light of events that were yet to come. Together they could almost be seen as fortune-tellers, predicting not what my future would bring so much as how I would respond to and deal with that future when it came.

SENTENCE 5. Sometimes my fears force me to . . . *pretend I'm not afraid.*
SENTENCE 63. I feel guilty when I . . . *don't enjoy sex.*

I finished all eighty-seven sentences that day. Feeling satisfied with my effort, I neatly placed the pages on a table near the front door. I would, I decided, carry the assignment with me the following week when I went to view the videotape of my first session. To put it in the mail would chance its getting lost. To carry it with me to my next session might imply that I had not attended to the assignment until the last moment. My date for the videotape viewing seemed the best time for giving Dr. Leonard this first of many written works.

I reread those two pages several times, checking for spelling errors, legibility, and grammar. I wanted my work to be perfect.

I reread Sentence 59 more than the others. Not because I saw imperfections, but because it gave me a feeling of peace and satisfaction. It reminded me of the sureness I felt about the road I had chosen for myself half a year ago in Chicago. It alleviated any guilt I experienced over moving my family out to the East Coast.

SENTENCE 59.   To me the future looks . . . *bright*.

I was wrong.

5

THE ◇ FOUNDATION

By my fourth session, I had left my husband. It was not a move riddled with conflict or trauma. It was a decision neither suggested nor discouraged by Dr. Leonard. It was simply the right thing to do.

"Are you in love with David?" Dr. Leonard asked in my third session.

"Of course I love him," I replied.

"That wasn't the question. Are you in love with him?"

I had never asked myself that question. Never. Yet I knew in a second what the answer was.

My marriage was not a bad one by conventional standards. There was no violence, no drinking, no habitual unemployment. There was nothing David did that I could point to and say that if it didn't stop, I was leaving.

We could enjoy each other's company, taking pleasure in discussions of ideas and contemporary issues at the dinner table or late at night in bed. We shared few common interests, but those we did drew us together. There was rarely a moment as close as those we spent following a concert. Rachmaninoff and Saint-Saëns could make us feel together what we were incapable of feeling for one another alone.

At worst, the marriage was vacant. Void of depth and romance, we were sleepwalking through the motions of being married. We argued over matters of a personal nature, and that was the only passion ever felt between us. There was little sex in our marriage, and what there was was worse than unsatisfying. It left me feeling empty, lonely, and crying into my pillow for something more.

David cared for me much the way a father might. Quick to reprimand me if I had erred, he was equally free with praise and rewards when I had done well. He found me not pretty or sexy, but "cute" and "precious," and called me "Kitten" when an expression or pose struck him particularly so. And if I could not sleep at night, he would make up wonderful fairy tales about The Kitten and The Tiger (the latter being a referent to him) to help me sleep.

He was not an unkind man, but the depth of his feelings and the degree of his sensitivity were severely limited. He had a reputation for being rude and crass. He did not intend to be so, he just knew no other way.

David was well educated. Not an intelligent man, he compensated with his breadth of knowledge. How much he knew often intimidated me as he assumed the role of my teacher. But how poorly he reasoned alienated me, as I experienced myself in a different world, unable to comprehend how he could ever survive in his.

My husband loved me. He loved things about me that no one else had even acknowledged existed. He found me intelligent, extremely so. He enjoyed my wit and sense of humor, and as a result, my company. He cared for me deeply and showed it. With words, with actions, with gifts, he made me feel loved. And I needed that.

I did not think about what I did or did not feel for David, other than wishing I found him attractive. He was gawky and not a handsome man. More amusing in appearance than appealing. But I knew, somewhere, that he was everything of which my mother would approve. He was well educated, ambitious, white, and Jewish—not necessarily in that order of importance. And so, still in search of her approval and still in search of a person who would love me, I married David.

The day on which I turned nineteen, David proposed and I accepted. From that day in November 1969, until our marriage in March 1970, I was sick to my stomach every single day.

"This nervousness is normal," my mother assured me. "Every bride-to-be feels this way." She said she had.

I clung to my mother's words like glue and waited for the day after the wedding to bring me relief. When the day after my wedding brought me only a flood of uncontrollable tears, my mother assured me that "every new bride cries like that the day after her wedding." Again, she said that she had. The relief never came.

I eventually settled into the marriage and my stomach eventually settled down. I dropped out of college and went to work as a receptionist. My husband went to work during the day and to graduate school at night. I learned how to cook and dutifully prepared elaborate dinners for my new husband. I came to count on my Steak Diane for self-esteem as much as I did my clean kitchen floor and spotless bathroom. I was learning to be a good wife.

With the easing of my stomach problems came a blanket of mild depression. I resigned myself to this existence and told myself that it was good. I saw my life as a role to be played out and looked to my mother for the model, even though it was a model I had intellectually rejected a long time ago.

Anxiety attacks interrupted the boredom of my life. As I reflected on the dreams I had once had, my mind was stirred and it let me know it with a pounding heart and sense of painful urgency.

I recalled my dreams to go to law school. I had wanted to be a lawyer ever since high school. Maybe even before that. I fantasized about being a lawyer; I read books about lawyers; I could envision my future only as a lawyer. A part of me was not letting me forget that.

"What made you give it up?" Dr. Leonard would ask me at a later time.

"I don't know, really. Part of it was that I didn't think I was smart enough," I answered.

"Who taught you that?"

"I don't know."

"Do you believe it?"

"I guess not," I replied.

"Somewhere you do," he answered. "And what's the other part?"

"Just a feeling inside that tells me I can't be anything important."

"Who taught you *that?*"

I thought back to a time when I was still a little girl. "Mommy!" I was calling with excitement as I ran to find her in the kitchen. I had made an important decision that I wanted to share. "Mommy," I said when I had found her, "I'm going to be something special when I grow up. I'm going to do something great!"

"No you won't!" she snapped back. "You'll grow up to be a damned housewife like the rest of us!"

"My mother," I told Dr. Leonard. "My mother."

"In more ways than you know," he answered knowingly and sympathetically.

It was the anxiety attacks and the worsening depression that first told me that my marriage to David might have been a mistake. I began to contemplate how I would feel divorced from David and single again.

It was at this time that I began vomiting again: every morning upon rising and sometimes straight through the day. I could not understand how my pending marriage to David had evoked the same psychosomatic symptoms as my consideration of divorce from him. Perhaps I was physically ill, it finally occurred to me, or allergic to the toothpaste, since mornings—right after brushing my teeth—seemed worse than any other time. Perhaps this was not psychosomatic at all.

43

I was flat on my back, my legs in the stirrups, and the gyne-cologist's hand well inside of me when he told me I was ten weeks pregnant. That, he chuckled, was the cause of my sick-ness. First I sobbed. Then I dismissed any further thoughts about divorce.

I tried not to think about the loneliness I felt in this mar-riage. I concentrated on adjusting to the prospect of spending the rest of my life with David and to my impending moth-erhood. And my depression deepened.

As caring and loving as David was with me during this period, I could not escape the feeling of doom. This was not what I had wanted for my life. More importantly, this was not how I believed it had to be. I was in my ninth month of preg-nancy when I told David of my intention to move to New York for therapy. With or without him, I had to go where I knew there was help. He loved me too much to let me go alone. When he said he would start looking for work out East, I tele-phoned Dr. Blumenthal.

"No," I said with certainty. "I am not in love with my hus-band." I went home from that session and told David I wanted a divorce.

As I set about freeing myself from past mistakes, I also spent a great deal of time building new relationships and strengthen-ing other old ones. Almost all of my friends now were patients of Dr. Leonard, united by a central theme: therapy with and respect for Lonnie Franklin Leonard. Not that we did not share any other values. We did. But those values that didn't involve our therapist usually involved Objectivism. My perspective was narrowing, my world was shrinking. Objectivism, Objectivists, and Objectivist Psychotherapy were becoming all I knew. And without being aware of it, I was both suffocating under and helping to propagate the rules that seemed to accompany my acceptance by other students of Objectivism.

Living as a "student of Objectivism" brought with it a whole set of rules and regulations. Sometimes these were deduced by the students themselves; other times, they could be found in the lectures and publications of Objectivists. *Objectivists,* as distin-guished from *students of Objectivism,* were those whom Ayn Rand had designated a graduate, of sorts, of her philosophy; one who was "sanctioned" to espouse or interpret her work. Allan Blumenthal received Ayn Rand's sanction. Lonnie Leonard re-ceived Allan Blumenthal's.

Whatever their source, there seemed to be rules of right and wrong for *everything* in Objectivism. There was more than just a right kind of politics and a right kind of moral code. There was also a right kind of music, a right kind of art, a right kind of interior design, a right kind of dancing. There were wrong books which we could not buy, and right ones which we should. Wrong books were written by "immoral" people whom we didn't want to support through our purchase; right books never were. There were plays we should not see, records we should not listen to, and movies we should not pay to watch. There were right ways to behave at parties, and right people to invite to them. And there were, of course, right psycho-therapists. And on everything, absolutely everything, one was constantly being judged, just as one was expected to be judging everything around him. And if one was not judging everything that was around him, one was judged on that, too. It was a perfect breeding ground for insecurity, fear, and paranoia.

My first exposure to this unsuspected practice among stu-dents of Objectivism came within weeks of my introduction to the social world that revolved around the philosophy. I was in-vited to attend a party. A party, to Objectivists, apparently meant something other than dancing, socializing, music, or laughter. This party and many that followed were discussions on topics like *epistemology, metaphysics, ethics,* or *politics.* That night's conversation turned to the political, and not being one to ever walk away from a good discussion or debate, I played devil's advocate. A week after the party, I received a letter from the party's hostess in which she "condemned" my behavior and informed me that the role of a devil's advocate was "immoral."

I was devastated. I had finally found other people who held

the same ideas as I, and I had blown it. I had behaved immorally. I was back to being alone because my new friends obviously knew more about this philosophy business than I did. And they knew I was a bad person. So bad, in fact, that I could never be invited back to their parties.

I recovered from that episode when I met a new group of students of Objectivism. I was more careful this time around, but apparently not careful enough. Whereas I was not condemned when I married David, several of our Objectivist friends "boycotted" our wedding. The grounds: Ellen did not have an established career. I didn't know about that rule, but apparently they did. David and I were judged accordingly, but not to the extent of being condemned.

By the time I was relocated in New York and acquainted with those people who had been living in the capital city of Objectivism, I had learned that there was little, if anything, that was exempt from moral judgment. One was at constant risk of losing all of one's friends. And if one lost these friends, one had lost the best in the world. They were trustworthy and honest. They were ambitious and intelligent. They were productive and moral. They were, after all, students of Objectivism.

In the beginning, Dr. Leonard's entourage of patients was no different from the larger circle of Objectivists I knew. If anything, they were even more extreme in that they added, to all of their virtues, growing mental health. They lived by all the rules and made judgments with the same self-righteousness. The difference, however, was that we had a real-life hero to emulate. Dr. Leonard represented himself as the healthiest man he knew, and urged us to look to him as our example.

"Don't you have any flaws?" I asked him early on.

"Well, if you see any, let me know. But I don't think you will," he answered.

So we did more than give him our respect and adoration. We gave him our loyalty. Unquestioningly.

We had heard, for example, that Dr. Leonard had expelled

from therapy a distant acquaintance of ours. We knew none of the particulars, only that he had been dismissed and was being shamefully secretive about the occurrence. No explicit judgments were made among my friends and myself, but the tone with which the matter was discussed conveyed as much as any words could have. Clearly, our acquaintance had done something immoral. Whatever his sin, be it a lie or an evasion, Dr. Leonard, in his vast scheme of justice, had determined this man unworthy of his treatment, time, and brilliance. There was, after all, a long line of people who wanted to improve, wanted to be happy, wanted to be perfectly healthy.

Any discomfort we may have felt over judging, albeit implicitly, a situation about which we had no facts, was overshadowed by the sense of moral self-righteousness we took from being among the group that was good enough to remain under his care.

Then, in the months soon after my first session with Dr. Leonard, he set about freeing us from the chains of Objectivist rules.

"He told me there was nothing wrong with seeing a baseball game or spending time on a Sunday afternoon watching football," one patient told me.

"He told me rock 'n' roll dancing was okay," another patient reported.

"Dr. Leonard says some of these things are 'optional' values and have no right or wrong," said one other.

Dr. Leonard was giving his patients permission to do some of the things they liked that Objectivism had intimidated them out of pursuing. This made him a "rebel" and a greater hero. He not only knew enough to understand the rules, he knew enough to understand why it was okay to break them without being immoral. He taught us that we had been chained to Objectivism, imprisoned by its laws without our awareness. He also told us that he could free us and we responded by being willing to follow him anywhere.

My own therapy during these first few months was both a time of growing trust in and growing uneasiness about Dr.

Leonard. The trust was a natural consequence of the disclosures that came with therapy, and the support and understanding that were delivered in return.

"But my therapist told me that it was a Freudian fantasy," I explained to him after telling him about the night in the maid's room with my father. I waited to see what he would say.

"That kind of psychological garbage was very prevalent around the time you're talking about—what was it, about five, ten years ago?"

"Yes," I answered with amazement, "the therapy was about seven years ago." I paused, and then asked, "You mean, you believe it happened? You believe it is reality I am recalling and not a fantasy?"

"Oh, it's reality," he replied with certainty. "It's reality."

He believed me. Just like that. I had been all prepared to defend my perceptions, recount the discussion I had had with my father at my psychiatrist's urging, and insist I knew what I was talking about. But he believed me. I didn't realize how important being believed on this issue was, until he believed me.

Any uneasiness I felt I attributed to my neurosis: a subconscious resistance to naming my problems, I told myself. In almost all situations that produced negative emotional reactions toward Dr. Leonard, I gave him the benefit of the doubt and myself the blame for unhealthy reactions. After all, he was the doctor and perfectly healthy, and I was the patient and not. This served to further undermine my trust in the validity of my own emotional responses, as well as the confidence in my ability to judge. It also increased my dependency on my therapist, as I came to substitute his opinions and advice for my own common sense.

Still my therapy was riddled with insecurities and doubts. For example, following a particularly productive session in which a conflict had been resolved or an emotion had been explored, Dr. Leonard would rhetorically ask: "With your problems, where else do you think you could get this kind of help?"

At times when I felt myself just beginning to get angry at him, he would similarly pose: "You have someplace else you can go?" His questions told me two things: how bad off he thought I was, and that no one but him could help me to change that. Together they evoked a strange combination of grateful entrapment.

Therapy was, for us all, the most important part of our lives and we were proud of it. A young crowd, most of us were just starting out. Incomes were generally low and financial struggles were taken in stride as a small price to pay for the better life that awaited us. Dr. Leonard was being paid with grocery money or better housing rent. Apartments were shared three ways, or tenement living was selected by those preferring to live alone. Meals for one day were stretched to fit two; some meals were skipped altogether. But no sacrifice was too great. It was, we agreed, the greatest value we could be pursuing.

Dr. Leonard's talents went beyond his ability to peer into our pasts and see the scars they had left. He did more than identify the source of injuries long since passed. He did more than sympathize, console, and care; more than probe, question, and listen. He lectured.

I had heard about his lectures even before starting my own therapy with him. My friends had marveled at the identifications Dr. Leonard had made in the field of psychology. He would, they continued to claim, revolutionize the entire profession with his contributions. How fortunate we all felt to be a part of this new frontier.

The lectures, as far as we could gather by comparing notes, were fairly standardized. The application of the contents of the lecture to one's own personal context might come later, but the lecture was delivered objectively and without reference to the patient hearing it.

These sessions were very different from the others. Instead of taking notes, Dr. Leonard used his pen for purposes of illustrating and diagraming his points. His tone changed from gentle, active listener, to self-impressed, authoritative orator. He tended to be much more impatient if an intellectual concept was not being grasped by the patient, than if a memory was being blocked.

Often the lectures consumed the entirety of the hour, if not more. It was necessary, if not expected, that notes would be taken by the patient during the viewing of the videotape for that session. Sometimes it was necessary for patients to see the tape two or three times in order to fully comprehend that day's lesson. He had a lecture on Hostility, on Values, on Careers, and on how to integrate the new ideas he was teaching us in place of the old ones of which we were trying to rid ourselves. But the lecture which was the most significant for me was the one on Romantic Love.

"Everybody is a certain percentage of somebody else's perfect partner," he began. "For example, any given man that you meet on the street, Ellen, might be five percent or one hundred percent of what you're looking for."

"What makes you so sure he might even be five percent?" I interrupted.

He was clearly annoyed. "He's got a pecker, doesn't he? That's got to be worth some percentage points!"

Responses like that taught me early on how to spot the times I was not suppose to question him—and there were many.

With aggravation in his voice, he continued the lecture. He restated his first point and proceeded.

"If a person is married to or dating another who is less than one hundred percent of what they ideally want in a partner, it is necessary to first name what percentage is actually being fulfilled—or conversely, what percentage is missing.

"Assume for the moment," he told me, "that a woman places her husband at eighty-five percent of what she really wants. She is missing fifteen percent.

"She should be looking for that fifteen percent," he said. "Not looking means that she is accepting less than what would make her totally happy."

Dr. Leonard explained that she could stay with her present

partner while continuing her search for the missing fifteen percent, but that this was second best to leaving her mate. Such a situation, he claimed, made it difficult for her to devote enough energy to her search.

It became easy to tell when patients in romantic relationships had received this part of the lecture. All of a sudden, they were measuring one another in terms of percentage points and either forming an open-marriage sort of relationship so as to free themselves for the search for the missing percentage, or dissolving their relationship altogether so as to find that perfect partner faster.

"Men are polygamous by nature," he continued to lecture, "but of women I am not so sure."

"How are you so positive about men?" I asked him.

"By looking at my own psychology," he replied. "Since I am the only perfectly healthy man I know, it is legitimate for me to draw on my own introspective material for research data. I am healthy and I am polygamous, therefore polygamy is most likely in the nature of men."

That brought him into a discussion of the sequence of events in a healthy romantic relationship.

"On the sequence of events that occur in a healthy romantic relationship, I have absolutely no doubts," he said. "Man has the primary role in a romantic relationship.

"A man can penetrate a woman whether she's ready or not, whether she's wanting or not. He needs to get and maintain an erection. She does not even have to be excited. So physiologically, he is the *primary actor.*

"A woman's sexual feelings come from her response to a man," he explained. "So the man becomes primary in a second way. She is dependent on him not only for sexual satisfaction, but for any sexual feelings at all."

This all led him to the conclusion that a romantic relation could exist with a woman loving, i.e., responding to and admiring a man, and the man just letting her love him. His pleasure would come from her showing him her love; hers would come from his letting her. No reciprocal response would be necessary. Not for quite some time.

At that time, my self-doubt allowed me to dismiss as neurotic any information about myself that contradicted his words, and my sexual naïveté and inexperience allowed me to accept the balance of my therapist's "facts" and conclusions. Many years after this time, however, I would come to know more about human sexuality through conversations with a girlfriend, which validated my own sexual nature, and through a special romantic relationship. Only then would I be able to judge this doctor's ignorance of female sexuality, and become incensed over the myths he had perpetuated.

He concluded with what appeared to be a remark of obvious truth.

"The better, healthier, more productive the man, the stronger the response from the healthy woman than to a man with lesser qualities. And a woman not responding to such a man when she sees him has a problem."

Only in hindsight did it become clear that the remark was designed to direct my *correct* response to him.

In revealing my past and finding his support and understanding, I felt my trust in Dr. Leonard growing. The priority I gave to his judgments over mine, the grateful entrapment I experienced over his remarks at a session's conclusion, and my unrelenting desire to become happy and perfectly healthy, transformed trust into dependency.

This trust and dependency that developed between January 6, 1972, and April 5 of that same year, laid the emotional foundation for what was to come. The lecture on Romantic Love provided its intellectual counterpart.

6

THE ◇ FIRST
ENCOUNTER

April 5, 1972

I arrived for the viewing of my videotape shortly before 8:00
P.M. On this particular occasion, I found the kitchen door
closed, which meant that the seven o'clock viewer was still inside. Moving toward the sofa to find a seat, I spotted another
patient waiting, as well. I knew that Dr. Leonard's seven o'clock
session was his last of the day; it would be ending shortly. Unless this patient had been scheduled for a session during the
doctor's dinner hour, two of us had been scheduled to see our
tapes at the same time. Worse yet, I thought, perhaps I had
come on the wrong day or at the wrong time.

Tapes that were scheduled to be seen at eight o'clock did not
interfere with Dr. Leonard's dinner. He took most of his evening meals in restaurants. Often, I was left alone in his apartment between eight and nine o'clock to view my tape while he
went out to eat. The kitchen, it seemed, was used much more
regularly for the "loony tunes," as we jokingly called them, than
it was for the preparation of meals.

At a bit past eight, the kitchen door opened and the occu-
pant of the viewing room departed. As the other patient and I
both rose, Dr. Leonard emerged from his last session of the day.

"I think a mistake has been made," I said to him. Then I prayed it wasn't mine.

"No," he replied with a friendly smile. "You," he said looking at the other patient, "go to the kitchen. You," he said looking at me, "follow me."

He led me to his office, where the machinery that had always been used to record my sessions was now going to be used to play one back to me. I liked this. The patient's chair in his office was far more comfortable than the barstool we used in the kitchen. And the environment itself was warmer and safer; this was the place of my therapy with Dr. Leonard.

There was also something childishly adventuresome about being in the back of Dr. Leonard's apartment after working hours, after dark. It did not feel unlike those rare occasions when my parents had permitted me to stay up past my bedtime so that I could mingle a few minutes with their party guests. The invitation, as insignificant as I could tell it was to them, made me feel special. It let me pretend for those five minutes that I was an equal; I, too, had been invited.

Dr. Leonard was trusting me to be alone in his office. He trusted me alone with his file cabinet, his folders of notes, his records. He had invited me, not the other patient, to enjoy the comfort of his office. Was I not somehow special? Could this not be taken as a sign of movement toward equality?

Not being familiar with the operation of this machine, I had Dr. Leonard begin the tape for me. Before leaving for dinner, he explained how to rewind the tape when I finished. The tape was playing, but I heard little of the first fifteen minutes. My mind was preoccupied with the feelings I had at just being there and with being allowed to be there. It amazed me how much of Dr. Leonard's presence I could feel in the office, even in his absence. I felt the same sense of security as when he had been seated across from me behind the desk offering me understanding and guidance. I felt the same comfort as when he had consoled me and dried my tears. I felt the same awe of his wisdom glancing at his books as when he had given me advice. The

54

associations held in that room were powerful. I did not draw from its power, I surrendered to it and depended on it. I relaxed in the chair knowing that no harm could come to me there.

It was after my attention returned to the tape that was still playing that I became aware of a gradual erosion of the contentment I had been experiencing. Contentment was suddenly being replaced with anxiety. I felt a growing urge to run home, not to the bus or to the train station, but all the way home to Yonkers. I knew I could have made the run in less time than it would have taken to wait for the train. Then I began to hyperventilate. I tried to watch the rest of the tape, but I was unable to focus on the television screen.

By the time the machine had completed its playback of my session, my condition had worsened. I gathered my notebook, pen, and purse, and headed for the office door without rewinding my tape, as we were always expected to do.

My feet and fingers had gone numb from the hyperventilating. My head was growing lighter, and my anxiety was increasing. So when I opened the door and found Dr. Leonard standing naked in the hall just outside his office, I did not stop to take notice, nor did I react with surprise or fear. I kept only one goal in mind and continued my rush to the front door of the apartment.

"Stop!" he ordered and begged at the same time. "You're in no condition to go home." He did not move from his spot in the hall.

Ignoring him, I grabbed my wrap which was hanging on a hook in the vestibule and left. A spring action on the door closed it behind me as I made my way to the elevator.

Still naked, save for a towel thrown over his shoulder, he followed me into the outer hall. There we stood at the elevator, me hyperventilating and him au naturel. He placed his left arm around me and, with his right arm on my elbow, led me back to his apartment.

"I want you to lie down," he said firmly but gently. He escorted me to the end of the hall, beyond his office, beyond the bathroom across from the office, and into his bedroom. He took me to the bed, where he maneuvered me first into a sitting position and then, lifting my legs off the floor, into a horizontal one. He sat, still naked, next to me.

"Breathe slowly," he instructed. He told me to concentrate on taking long deep breaths, counting off each one in time. "If you don't control your breathing, I'll have to get you a paper bag to breath into," he warned.

My breathing began to stabilize.

"I was on my way into the shower when you came out of my office. I'm going to leave you alone for a few minutes while I finish what I started out to do a few minutes ago. Okay?"

When he returned less than ten minutes later, he was carrying a drink in one hand and his towel in the other. And he was still naked.

"Would you like some of my drink?" he offered.

"No. No thank you," I replied.

Then he left to dispose of his towel.

When he returned for the second time, he ordered me to remove my blouse as he produced a stethoscope.

"I can't remove my clothes in front of you," I replied shyly.

"First of all," he said sternly, "I am a doctor. I was doing physical examinations long before I ever practiced psychiatry. Second of all, don't you trust me?"

I slowly removed my blouse and he checked my vital signs.

"Who's watching your baby?" he inquired.

"David is staying with him while I'm here."

"You can't go home tonight. I'll phone him and let him know you'll be staying with me. It's the phone number in your record, right?"

"I'm fine now," I insisted. "I'm sure I can make it home okay."

He wasn't listening to me; he was leaving the bedroom to phone David from his office.

When Dr. Leonard joined me again, he was carrying a refilled glass out of which he again offered me a taste. The offer was unsettling for me, as it had been the first time it was made. It displayed a familiarity between us that I did not recognize. It was a familiarity that had not even existed during the half hour or so of Dr. Leonard's nudity which preceded this second offer.

"No. Thank you, but no," I answered while I thought over this matter.

He made no effort to cover or explain his nakedness. He was not embarrassed. He was not even concerned. He acted no differently than had he been fully attired in business clothes. And when I considered his nude jaunt into the outer hallway, I wondered if he knew he was naked at all.

But the drink, that was different. The drink could not be explained as a moment of coincidental timing; it was a moment being deliberately created. He did not act as if he held no drink in his hand the way he acted like he was not without clothes. It was not a doctor and patient accidentally meeting at an inopportune moment. It was not a doctor and patient at all. Doctors do not offer their patients a drink in bed.

"No," I repeated, "no, I really think I should be going home." My discomfort was showing, and I was embarrassed that it was.

"Okay. I just thought it might help you to relax," he explained.

Relax? Had the offer been a medical suggestion? Was the purpose of the drink strictly medicinal? Of course it was! How could I have felt that it was anything else? I was ashamed at having been so unnerved.

Instead of the drink, he gave me a sleeping pill. While I rested, Dr. Leonard breezed in and out of his bedroom. He moved between his office and where I was relaxing, periodically asking how I was.

He remained naked. His incredible nonchalance told me that psychologically healthy people are not embarrassed by casual nudity. Only neurotics, like me I supposed, were. I must not show it, I told myself. Then I gave myself a standing order to fix that part of my psychology.

He remarked during one of his brief returns to the bedroom that he did not mind taking care of me, but that he would not allow his generosity to interfere with his normal routine. He would not alter his life-style; I would have to fit myself into it.

I assumed that this was meant in reference to his lack of attire. I listened to what he said with the same unquestioning acceptance that I did almost everything he told me.

At eleven o'clock, he turned on the television to watch the news. I was still in the same position in which he had placed me an hour and a half earlier. He sat at the foot of the bed. He chattered during the broadcast, commenting on the reporting of the day's events and on the quality of journalism, or lack of it, on that particular network. Then, with obvious contempt in his voice, he questioned what one of the female reporters was doing on television.

"She's too ugly for a visual medium," he proclaimed. "There's only one way a woman like that makes it onto television." He paused, then added, "On second thought, who would want her *that* way?"

I could not respond to what I was hearing, for in it I was reliving every cruel moment in my childhood when I was taunted for being too ugly, too fat, or too tall. That pain not only paralyzed any response I may have thought about delivering, but I knew it had to be skewing my judgment, as well. I could not trust my reaction to be rational, therefore I could not trust it to be right, either. I said nothing.

At the end of the news, he brought me a second sleeping pill and a glass of water. After replacing the glass in the bathroom when I had finished, he crawled into bed and announced it was time to sleep.

Sleep in the same bed? We were going to sleep in the same bed together? I didn't know whether I should feel scared or special. I moved to the far edge of the bed with my arms straight down by my side, closed my eyes and said good night.

"Are you going to sleep like that?" he asked.

"Like what?"

"With all those clothes on?" he answered.

Now I knew. I was scared.

"I'm very comfortable. Really."

"Take them off," he ordered gently.

"No, I'm fine. I really am."

"Don't you trust me, Ellen?"

"Of course I do," I responded with defensiveness. "It's not that."

"Don't you enjoy the feelings of closeness we have during your therapy sessions?" he asked.

"Yes, of course I do. But what's the connection?"

"If you enjoy that closeness during your sessions, you should try to feel that closeness here. Now."

Panic began to take over and great effort was needed to hide it.

"I really am comfortable," I reassured him. "I sleep this way all the time." I lied.

"If you really trust me, I want you to show it."

"Couldn't I just show it down to my slip?" I giggled nervously to indicate that I was only half serious.

"Are you ashamed of your body?" he asked.

"No."

"Then it's that you don't trust me?"

"No. I mean, no, that's not it."

"You don't want to be close with me?"

"That has nothing to do with it. Why can't I feel close with my clothes on?" I asked him.

He did not answer. He delivered an ultimatum instead.

It was not the ultimatum itself that told me I had no choice in this matter, it was the tone of impatience, disapproval, and aggravation with which it was delivered.

"If you don't remove your clothes, you cannot sleep in this bed." Then he added, "And at this hour, you have nowhere else to go."

The issue was clearly important. I just could not tell if it was important to him, or if he thought as my therapist that it should be important to me. And I felt myself on the brink of being judged.

"Push yourself," he instructed. "Just force your way through those fears."

He did not watch me while I stripped. And he did not look at me after I had. I covered myself with the sheet, as there was no blanket.

"That's better," he seemed to say to his pillow. Then to me he said, "If you're not asleep by one o'clock, wake me."

"Okay," I promised. "Good night."

"Good night," he mumbled, as if he was already falling off to sleep.

I lay frozen and naked in my therapist's bed. I tried to relax with soothing thoughts:

This really is quite beautiful, you know. Here I am lying naked with the person who knows me better than anyone else in the world. This is open and trusting and close. This is good.

And what a compliment this is. He cares enough about me to take me in for the night, give me advice, offer me a drink, give me sleeping pills, and share his bed.

I should feel ashamed for resisting him, for being so scared, and for making him work so hard during his off-hours.

Then I thought to myself, after these words had been turned over and over in my mind, that I should feel ashamed of myself for still being so scared.

I could not relax. I could not sleep. I vacillated between uncertainty about the situation and force-fed reassurances. When, by one o'clock, sleep seemed impossible, I checked to see that the sheet totally covered me and I woke my doctor.

"It's one o'clock," I whispered. "I'm still not sleeping."

He rose quickly from the bed and went to his dresser drawer. Then he went to the bathroom sink, where he filled my glass with water. He returned with two sleeping pills and the glass.

"But that's four sleeping pills in less than four hours," I reminded him.

"It's okay," he reassured me.

I took the pills and he returned to bed. As the minutes passed, I knew I would sleep now. I grew sleepy and began to feel safety, not fear, in the stillness that once again was settling over the bedroom. I could hear Dr. Leonard's breathing; it was deep and rhythmic. His body did not move except for the rising and falling of his back as he inhaled and exhaled. The traffic noises rose from the streets like a distant, muted symphony, bringing comfort in the reminder of a reality that extended beyond the walls of therapy and my anxieties. I felt groggy. I felt peaceful.

I could not have been sleeping for more than a few minutes when I awoke to the awareness of movement in the bed. I opened my eyes to find Dr. Leonard on his hands and knees, staring into my face.

Before a word could be spoken, he jumped on top of me and wrapped his arms tightly around me.

"Fight me," he ordered in a whisper.

"What? What?" I stuttered. "What are you doing?"

"Fight me!" he ordered louder than the first time.

He was pressing against me tighter now, squeezing his arms around my back.

"I don't want to fight with you, Dr. Leonard."

He moved off me just long enough to jerk the sheet back. He immediately resumed his position in between my legs. He pressed my shoulders to the bed and taunted, "Don't you know how to wrestle?"

"No. No, I don't," I cried.

"Nobody taught ya, huh? Well, you can do it. Just struggle. Just fight."

I did not understand this. I did not understand what he was doing or what he wanted from me. Was this some kind of psychology test? Was this an example of how healthy men expressed romantic interest? Why was he doing this to me?

With fierceness in his voice, he repeated his whispered order. "Wrestle with me, damn it! Can't you fight at all?"

With that, he moved up against me, pressing his erection against my vagina, but not entering me. "NOW FIGHT!" he shouted. "Try to get away!"

I started to fight, not in obedience but in terror. The harder I struggled to free myself, the harder he tightened his grip on me.

"Go on," he urged. "That's it. Fight!"

I fought harder. His penis still did not enter me, nor was it removed from its threatening position. He seemed clearly to be enjoying this display of restrained power.

"Please let me go," I pleaded.

He released his grasp on me and moved off my body. Leaning back on his forearms and elbows, he looked at me and smiled. And I knew it wasn't over.

He took me by the waist and rolled me over on top of him so that my back was pressed against his chest. He cupped his hands over my breasts and whispered again, "Fight me, Ellen. Fight."

Maybe, I thought, he thinks that I am somehow enjoying this. "I don't want to fight with you, Dr. Leonard," I told him. "I'm really not enjoying this." I tried to say it calmly and without signs of the panic I was really in.

He fondled my breasts harder until I told him how much he was hurting me.

"Then fight to free yourself," he instructed.

I stopped struggling. I stopped begging. I stopped crying. My body went limp on his, my arms falling to my sides and my head rolling to one side. "I can't," I whispered in confused defeat. "I can't stop you."

With that, he rolled me onto my back and resumed his superior position with which the episode had begun. "I wanted you to wrestle with me," he said angrily. "I thought you would understand what I wanted, but you didn't. I thought you would know what to do, but you didn't."

There was a judgment being made here. I had fallen short of his expectations of me. I did not understand where or how. I only knew that I was being judged as psychologically less perfect, less at his level, than he had judged me before. I had not been able to understand him, and that was clearly a symptom of a deficiency in my psychology.

"I don't understand any of this, Dr. Leonard. What did I do wrong?"

My question and the feelings were painfully reminiscent of my past. I had never expected to relive those kinds of experiences with my Objectivist psychotherapist. That I was, gave me the feeling that the world was disintegrating.

"You'll understand in time," he said without any tone of comfort. "You'll understand when you're healthy." His answer was abrupt, and his irritation told me not to press the matter any further.

He rolled onto his side, putting his back to me. I began to sob uncontrollably. Once again, I was feeling confused and guilt-ridden for unknown crimes in a world that I should have been able to count on as clear, understandable, and accepting.

I crawled off his bed and found my way to the farthest corner of the room where I sat naked on the floor and cried as quietly as I could, for fear of disturbing his sleep.

Mommy may have been right, after all, I concluded in the darkness of Dr. Leonard's bedroom. There was something wrong with me, something that kept me from understanding the healthy people around me. My confusion *was* a consequence of my own flawed psychology. How else could I explain these same feelings that I thought had ended when I left my mother's home. How else, other than to place blame on everyone around me: my mother, my father, and now Dr. Leonard? It could not be, I reasoned. After all, this was an Objectivist psychotherapist. He was a person of rationality, reason, and perfect mental health. My evaluation of him was totally unlike that of my mother.

No, I thought, if I am incapable of comprehending the behavior I witnessed tonight, then the problem surely lies within me.

With the rising of the sun, I felt the risks to be less outside than inside Dr. Leonard's apartment. I dressed and left for Grand Central Station, certain that I had not disturbed him since leaving his bed.

This time when I approached the front door, I was not hyperventilating. I was not numb from too much oxygen and I was not light-headed. This time, I was dazed, exhausted, and nauseated. My head was throbbing and I continued to cry sporadically and uncontrollably. I felt that the whole world had gone mad. More accurately, that I had.

His words rang in my ears: that I would understand when I became healthy. Given my tormenting confusion, his consolation was more of an indictment on my present state of mental health than it was reason for hope. And he had, I reasoned, good cause for such an indictment, for I had not been able to understand the great Dr. Leonard. Worse yet, I had been scared by him.

I had not been able to show him easily, naturally, how much I trusted him; I could still feel the embarrassment at having removed my clothes. I had not understood what he had wanted or what I had been expected to do. I had understood nothing. Absolutely nothing.

Some day, I promised myself, I will be healthy enough to understand what happened last night.

7

ON◇BECOMING FEMININE

April 12, 1972

As my digestive system had always been the clearest barometer of my states of mind, so it was following the night I spent in Dr. Leonard's bedroom. Nausea and vomiting, stomach cramps and diarrhea, these were my constant reminders that Dr. Leonard thought I was too ill to understand the events of that fateful night. Further, they reminded me that I was not capable of coping with them, either.

I felt guilty and anxious the week between my viewing in his office and my next session. I needed help. That automatically translated into: I needed Dr. Leonard.

I didn't feel the turmoil constantly. The time spent caring for and playing with my son took me to another place where Dr. Leonard couldn't touch. Whether it was my need to escape or my son's ability to make me exclusively his during our time together, or both, I am not certain. But when his nap time came or he was put down for the night, my mood and mind would swing back to the night in Dr. Leonard's bedroom.

"I'm experiencing extreme mood changes," I told him during our session. "I can be high and happy and talking baby talk with my son in one minute, and crying, confused, and anxious the next.

"I feel so confused and guilty over what happened here. I have constant diarrhea, and sometimes I vomit, too."

"You'll feel better as you come to understand what I wanted," he explained.

"Well, that's sort of what I was hoping you could tell me now. I really need to know and I don't think my stomach will get any better until I do," I told him.

"You'll understand in time."

"But I want to know now. I have to know now."

"You'll understand when you become healthy. Then, no explanation will be needed."

I thought a moment, looking for a new approach that would make him tell me what I needed to know.

"Well, then, tell me what I did that made you so angry," I implored.

"That wasn't anger," he responded.

"What was it?" I asked with surprise.

He refused to say.

"When you come to understand what I wanted that night, Ellen, you'll be able to understand my reaction to you.

"When that time arrives in your life," he continued, "you will be the one who will be angry for passing up such an opportunity."

"When will that time come?"

"Whenever it is that you understand," he said with impatience.

"But I need answers now!"

"What answers do you want?" he asked in a challenging tone. "What answers do you want me to give you?"

"Tell me what you were expecting of me that night," I insisted.

"You'll understand that when you're healthier."

"Why were you so—upset afterward?" I pressed on.

"When you understand the answer to your first question, you'll have an answer to your second," he replied.

I was getting nowhere. I decided to pose a new question.

"Why me?"

He was disturbed at my asking it.

"I won't answer that. Besides, you shouldn't need to know," he answered.

"What?" I was not sure I had heard him correctly.

"Think about it on your own time," he said, trying to wrap up this conversation. "You have enough information to figure it out. All I'll say is that it should have been enough for you to be there."

When I finally gave up my efforts to press him into a conversation that he apparently did not want to have, he closed the subject by apologizing for having judged my psychology further along than it actually was.

"For that, I'll take responsibility," he offered. "I had thought you were more sexually mature and more feminine than you turned out to be. A healthy woman would have known what to do. At the very least, she would have found me sexually attractive."

With that, he insisted we move on to other topics "more suitable for a therapy session." He asked me what else was happening in my life.

"My mother and father are back in my life," I informed him.

"Well, that's a big change. How did that happen?"

"I called my father," I told him.

"How did the conversation go?" he asked.

"Terrific. I mean, he really sounded happy to hear from me. I don't think he knew what my mother had said to me on the phone last year. I mean, we didn't talk about it or anything, but he sure didn't sound like a parent who didn't want to see his daughter anymore. He was real upset to hear about my separation, though. That was rough on him."

"What about your mother?" he asked.

"With my father so happy to hear from me, I don't think my mother can hold onto her original position," I answered.

We continued like this until Dr. Leonard notified me that

we were out of time. When he rose from behind his desk, I quickly delivered my last comment for the day.

"I just want you to know that I think you are sexually exciting," I told him. I hoped his new evaluation of me would not remain so low. I hoped he would begin to see me again as a feminine woman. In the meantime, I would work hard on feeling the truth of my words and on becoming a perfectly healthy female.

In the weeks following that session, I played his words over and over in my head. Was I unfeminine because I did not really find him sexually exciting? Was I immature because I could not understand what he wanted? Was I neurotic because I needed to know why he had picked me?

I tried, in the sessions that followed, not to bring the issue up *too* often. The topic aggravated him terribly, and my efforts accomplished nothing. I found myself complaining about more stomach problems, and we looked for causes of this pain during much of my hour every other week—causes other than the true one.

It was his evaluation of me, rather than the event out of which it came, that weighed most heavily on my mind. I could not help but accept Dr. Leonard's judgment of what my behavior meant that night, and I vowed to work hard on correcting that part of me.

"How do you feel about me as a man?" he asked me sometimes in session.

"You're the best man I know," I would tell him. I believed it.

"How does that make you feel as a woman, Ellen?" he would then ask.

"It makes me feel sexual," I would tell him.

I knew it was a lie, but I knew it was the right answer. It always made him nod and smile so knowingly.

"Can you say that another way? Can you tell me *where* you feel it?" he would ask.

Usually I could not say what I knew he wanted to hear. Other times, I would reply, "In my vagina."

He would smile approvingly.

I was waiting one afternoon for a four o'clock session when Dr. Leonard entered the living room from the back hall. It was still his lunch hour and he had no patient with him. It was too early for my session to begin, and I wondered why he had come out.

"It's not time yet," I informed him.

"How would you like to rub my back? It's been bothering me lately."

Though his request made me uneasy, the manner in which he asked it, not to mention past discussions, told me that I should want to very much. He asked it with such matter-of-factness that I did not dwell on my discomfort.

"Okay," I answered, trying to sound equally casual in my reply. I waited for him to be seated next to me on the sofa when he disappeared into the hall from where he had come.

"Are you coming?" he called from the back of the apartment.

I remained glued to the edge of the couch while I tried to decide what I should do. Before a decision could be reached, he returned to the edge of the hall where he stuck his head around the corner and said, "Come on, I'm waiting for you." And he disappeared again.

I slowly rose and, as if I were being drawn in slow motion by some power outside myself, I found my way to his bedroom.

He was lying face down on the middle of his bed. He was naked. His head was turned away from the entrance to the bedroom. Aware of my presence at the door, he told me where his back hurt and how he liked it rubbed.

I took a seat on the edge of the bed and stretched to reach his shoulders. As I massaged his neck and upper back, he made no movements, no sounds. Several minutes passed like this, and then the silence was interrupted.

"Straddle my back," he ordered.

"That wouldn't be comfortable," I explained in defense of my inaction.

"It has to be more comfortable than how you're sitting now," he explained.

"No, it really wouldn't."

He did not argue. Instead, he quickly rolled over, looking first at me to see that I caught his eye, and then at his penis. He did not speak. He did not wait for me to speak.

He took my left hand and wrapped its fingers around his erection. With his hand guiding mine, he moved my hand up and down just a few times. Suddenly, he withdrew his hand from mine and ejaculated.

I was no longer nervous or scared. I was numb. Even as he complimented me on how feminine I was becoming, I could not feel anything. I was, at most, relieved that he was pleased with me.

"Next time you'll have to learn to cover it so we don't make such a mess," he said noncritically as he jumped off the bed.

"You don't have to return to the living room; you can wait for me in my office," he called from the master bathroom.

"May I ask you about what just happened?" I asked him as my session began.

His good mood immediately changed. "We were being close," he explained, already showing his impatience. "Can't you handle that?"

"Of course I can handle closeness, but I don't understand what the sex means."

"Don't you love me? Don't you trust me? Don't you enjoy being open with me?" He was clearly aggravated now.

"Yes, of course," I replied, for no other answer was possible.

"Then?" he asked as if to indicate that no further discussion was necessary—or permitted.

I should have known enough by then to take my cue from his tone of voice. And I should have been able to tell that any further questions would have been pushing too far. But I pressed on.

"Is this some kind of therapy, some kind of experimental therapy you're doing with me?"

He rose slowly from behind his desk, his eyes locking mine. His face went taut and his body rigid. He leaned on the palms of his hands so as to get as close to me as possible while remaining buffered by the desk.

"What—kind—of person—do—you—think— I—am?" he asked slowly, deliberately, and with great anger.

My confusion and need to understand were instantly replaced with fear. I had, indeed, pushed too hard, pressed too far. And I had asked the wrong question.

"Answer me!" he demanded after a few seconds had passed.

"I'm sorry. I really am." I meant it. "I was only grasping at straws. In my need to understand, I was willing to consider any answer, even the most absurd. I really didn't think it was therapy. I just wanted to make sure."

He stood erect now. Extending his left arm straight out to his side and pointing to the office wall that was shared by the master bedroom on the other side, he said, "*That* is one thing . . ."—moving his left hand straight down, pointing to his desk—he continued, ". . . and *this* is another."

I told him I understood, but I did not.

During the weeks and months that followed, it became necessary for me to find my own explanations for the events of my brief past with Dr. Leonard. I told myself that I was obviously special to my therapist. I had been singled out as worthy of his affections and deserving of his precious time outside of work. This was not a difficult conclusion to reach, as we both shared a philosophy that taught the importance of selectivity, discrimination, and respect in sex. In the context of those guidelines and "rules" of Objectivism, this perfect man had chosen me to share his time, bed, and body. That *had* to mean something.

That I was unable to respond to him was symptomatic of an underlying neurosis, I reasoned. It had to be, for any healthy woman would have responded freely and fully to this ideal man.

I could not risk angering him or alienating him with any improper management of the situation, for once I attained his level of mental health, I would be grateful for his attention and anxious to return it with meaning and feeling.

He was the hero in the story of my life, waiting patiently for the day when I could worship him fully. And I grew to appreciate his patience, as well as the compliment implied in the invitations to his bedroom.

But whereas this rationale helped to guide my behavior with Dr. Leonard, it was a different process that carried me through the routine of my days outside of his apartment.

I could not have conversed with friends about topics other than the one that was really on my mind, nor provided love and care for my baby with undivided attention, nor shopped for groceries, paid the bills, or cleaned the apartment, had I not begun to compartmentalize the upset of my relationship with Dr. Leonard from the rest of my life. Initially, I would have to force his image and all my lingering questions out of my mind. Whether I was bathing my son or scouring a sink, if Dr. Leonard came to mind, I would force him out of awareness and focus all the harder on my activity of the moment. Then this process became automatic. I didn't have to work at eliminating him from my thoughts; he simply disappeared. And eventually, he stopped creeping into areas where he didn't belong.

But when I was alone, and always the night before a session, he entered my thoughts and the anxiety became unbearable.

By the time I boarded the train the morning of my session, I was emotionally wrought and primed for the intense work that was expected of me during my hour with him. I boarded the train on the verge of tears, half anxious to see my doctor to get help from falling apart and half scared to see him for reasons I told myself were just signs of my deep neurosis. I always needed extra travel time for my frequent visits to the bathroom, as my diarrhea had worsened. And I was exhausted from not sleeping the night before. I entered Dr. Leonard's office a wreck waiting to happen.

Dr. Leonard seemed pleased at how easily my tears were produced, and how *on the surface* my pain seemed to be. My therapy became a combination of artificial efforts on my part to search for a cause of this anxiety other than the one I knew it to be, and compassionate guidance from my therapist over the causes that he came to name as the real culprits. The truth could not be identified by him, because his focus precluded consideration of it, and it could not be named by me, because my focus was now dictated by fear.

Dr. Leonard, nevertheless, handled this time with seeming patience and understanding. He dried my tears, reassured me when I doubted my sanity, and hugged me when I felt lost and frightened. The latter he did not only to provide comfort, but to help me resolve feelings of abandonment and loneliness, which I carried with me from the past. And as he held me and rocked me, he would whisper words of encouragement.

"Feel those little girl feelings," he would say softly. "Go with those feelings and see where they take you."

Such kindness and gentleness, albeit in response to relatively unimportant matters, nourished my admiration of and reaffirmed my trust in him.

Occasionally, I ventured forth to make new inquiries of him, but each time I did I incurred his wrath. From the same source that gave protective embraces and parental guidance, I believed I saw the capacity for tremendous violence. Sometime later, I would witness an incident that would prove me right. It was, intuitively, my safety I protected when I ceased asking questions. Only I did not know it at the time.

Nude jaunts became common practice for Dr. Leonard as he greeted his first morning and first after-lunch patients in this manner. Only female patients, however, were privy to this spectacle.

Women discussed their eyewitness accounts with lightness and casualness at small parties or gatherings. It became common knowledge that Dr. Leonard appeared naked before a select group of females, all of whom came to feel complimented by their inclusion. At first, I was surprised to hear the topic being discussed in public. But I came to accept the conversations, and participated in them, just as I had learned to accept his naked welcomes—with the same nonchalance as he and his other patients did.

I spent much of my time during these weeks in spring and summer *adjusting*. I was adjusting to sex with my therapist of what I thought was a bizarre nature. I was adjusting to not getting answers to my questions. I was adjusting to a psychotherapy that put certain topics off-limits. I was adjusting to seeing my therapist nude when he opened his front door to me. I was also adjusting to other women being greeted the same way, and to their apparent comfort at being so. Little could I comprehend at the time that this was not adjustment at all. It was forcing out of mind all of the unanswered conflicts whenever they emerged and swallowing the feelings of doubt, discomfort, and fear that accompanied them. But I believed I was getting better.

It was nearing summer when Dr. Leonard offered me a job as his maid. I had told him in a previous session of the financial strain I was experiencing as a result of therapy. Even the train tickets and babysitting expenses were draining me. The offer did not strike me as unusual so much as it did generous and kind. I was grateful for the favor I felt he was granting me.

He instructed me to come to his apartment on Fridays, the one day a week when he scheduled no regular sessions. He would pay me twenty-five dollars plus car fare for six hours of heavy-duty cleaning, the kind that his cleaning lady was too old to do. I took the job.

My chores on the first day of work included polishing the plumbing pipes under the sink and toilet, scraping the bathroom tiles of any excess grout, and vacuuming the carpets. The last was to be done not with a power attachment, but with the cylinder tube nozzle attached to the cannister.

"You've got to get on your hands and knees and suck up an inch or so of carpet like this." And he demonstrated.

He said that, if done properly, the job should take several hours to complete. Then he explained which direction he wanted the pile to lay in when I was finished. He ran his hand one way over the gold plush and said that this was *not* how he wanted to see it. He ran his hand in the opposite direction and told me to take note of the shade difference; that was how he wanted it.

He checked up on me periodically, pointing out an inch here and an inch there that did not lay in the right direction. He carefully inspected the bathroom pipes, as well, getting on the floor to inspect the quality of the shine.

"They must shine," he said, emphasizing the word *must*. That was the whole purpose of the job.

I finished my vacuuming and polishing by one-thirty and he the work he was doing in his office at the same time. He came into the hall where I was disassembling the vacuum cleaner and told me to leave the machine where it was and follow him. He headed for his bedroom.

He got on top of the bed, fully dressed, and patted the spot next to him where he wanted me to sit. He did not tell me where his back hurt, nor give me instructions on how to touch him, nor guide my hand to his penis. Instead, he took both my hands in his and he talked to me. He talked to me for a long time.

First he talked about how wonderful it is to be open and close with someone. I had heard this all before in here, but it felt different this time. This time, he had his clothes on.

Then he began to talk about himself. His medical schooling was done at the University of Arkansas, he said. I knew that already from the degree hanging in his office. He had attended the university from 1955 to 1959. He went on to explain that he had interned at the U.S. Navy Hospital in San Diego, and from there he went to the U.S. Navy School of Aviation Medicine in Pensacola, Florida, where he trained to become a U.S. Flight Surgeon. He seemed not to have disliked his experience with the Navy, as he shared several stories about those days with warmth and humor.

He then spoke briefly of his days in residency at Bellevue Hospital in New York. Those years, between 1966 and 1969, seemed not to be remembered with the same affection. Criticizing much of what he had witnessed in those with whom he had worked, he moved on to lighter topics.

He worked for a brief time as a consultant in psychiatry for IBM, but the experience apparently did not warrant any further discussion. From there, he had proceeded to build the successful private practice which he had that day.

He spoke about his two unsuccessful marriages. The first resulted in two sons. The boys lived in Arkansas with their mother, about whom he had very little to say. His second marriage was to a physician in New York City and had, he said, been a mistake from the beginning. It lasted less than a year.

Dr. Leonard held Dr. Blumenthal responsible for the failure of his second marriage. He said that Dr. Blumenthal and Objectivist Psychology in general did not have a real grasp of the essential issues concerning romantic relationships. Dr. Blumenthal, he explained, had been his mentor in the field of Objectivist Psychology, and the ideas that Dr. Leonard learned there had become his standard for his second marriage. The ideas had been mistaken; thus so was the marriage.

He told me he had ended up in New York City strictly by chance after his service in the Navy. He had flipped a coin. He had not been able to decide between the East Coast and the West. One was assigned heads, the other tails. Such was his method of decision.

He digressed and talked about his mother and father, speaking harshly about the latter. He relayed stories out of his childhood and some from not so long ago concerning his familial relationships. And then he stopped talking and just held onto my hands. He leaned back and closed his eyes.

I felt closer to him in this moment than I ever had before. I was not scared. I was not even nervous. And I had stopped second-guessing what he might do next. He had opened up to me and that made me feel enormously special to him. He had told me things that were private and which he had specified were not for public information. He trusted me. And in this very peaceful moment, I trusted him, too.

He opened his eyes now and looked at me. He released one of my hands and placed the other over his trousers where I could feel his erection.

"That's how it feels when it gets excited," he said. "Would you like to see it?"

He was talking to me as if this were my first sexual experience. He spoke to me almost as if I were a child. I did not answer him. I knew my answer would not matter.

After he removed his clothes, he placed my hand on his chest and told me to move it lightly over his body so that my fingers would almost tickle him. He guided my hand every inch of the way: first his chest, then his calves, then his thighs, and then his penis. He continued moving my hand for me, but gave me verbal instructions anyway. It was almost as if he were talking to himself. After he ejaculated, he did not touch me. He even released the hand which he had been holding for so long.

He did not ask me to leave right away. Instead, he invited me to join him in the bathtub, which I declined. When he returned from his bath, he took a seat on the white chair against the wall and called me over to him. He told me to sit on the floor at his feet.

Now he took my hands again and spoke more about openness and closeness. It was not any different from the talk earlier that afternoon or any of the others earlier that year. I could not tell, though, if he really wanted me to understand the points he was making, or if he did not remember having told me all of this before. It didn't really matter; I would not have stopped him anyway.

He paid me for the six hours I had been hired to work. I declined the cash, but he argued that he had asked me to re-serve those six hours and that I should be paid for them regardless of whether or not they were used. I felt like I was being paid for sexual services rendered, not cleaning services, and I told him so. He laughed.

"That's ridiculous," he said. Then he excused himself abruptly. He was, he said, in a hurry to move on with his day.

The frequency of such encounters increased over the summer. I was invited to stay after one o'clock sessions which ended at the commencement of his lunch hour. I was asked into his bedroom if I arrived just a few minutes before a four o'clock session or videotape viewing. The same was true for the ten o'clock hour, the first working hour of his day. And I was invited to spend several nights with him. There was no regularity, no predictability to the encounters. There was only frequency.

The mood of the sex between us never changed. He never kissed me, never caressed me, never held me. He showed no interest in my pleasure. He claimed, instead, that all my pleasure would come from pleasing him.

"Some day," he told me, "when you are totally feminine, you will be able to climax just by watching me motion you toward me with the flexing of my index finger."

So I accepted his instructions in bed without question—and without pleasure. And I strove to become the feminine woman he described.

A time came that summer when he stopped being satisfied with my masturbating him, though when I once asked him why he had never asked to have intercourse with me, he replied: "You have not earned that sanction yet, Ellen." I had, however, earned the sanction of fellating him.

He instructed me, again, on what to do to him. And once he introduced fellatio into our encounters, he rarely asked for anything else. He moved my face to where he wanted it and held it there while verbalizing his desires. And when it was over, he would compliment me on my increasing femininity and tell me how beautiful I was to watch. He approved, and I was glad.

78

8

PROBATION

His behavior grew increasingly incomprehensible as the summer wore on. Lapses of memory and episodes of confusion marked a noticeable departure from his usual lucidity.

Once, for example, upon entering his bedroom following a session, I saw an open cosmetic bag on the dresser. It contained a woman's toiletries and makeup. He had never explicitly told me that he had no other women in his life, but I had assumed, for some reason, that he would have informed me had that not been the case. He had told me about the status of his separation from his second wife, as if that should be of concern to me. I assumed that the presence of a new woman should have been of equal interest to me.

"Whose is that?" I asked with more curiosity than accusation. After all, we had no understanding between us, and he was, I recalled, polygamous by nature.

"I don't want to discuss this again," he replied.

"Again? When did we discuss this before?" I asked.

He repeated his refusal to discuss the matter, and added that once should be enough.

"But we've never discussed this." I wondered, was I losing my mind?

Half in amazement and half in anger, he proclaimed that we had just had a lengthy discussion about this new woman several weeks earlier. I denied that we had had any such conversation, for surely I would have recalled it. But he was equally adamant as we argued the point outside the bedroom.

"I think we should work on your faulty memory in therapy," he said. "It's suggestive of what you do with information you do not want to hear."

But I remained fixed in my conviction that this discussion to which he referred had never occurred between us. So he reluctantly "repeated" himself.

He had, he said, found a woman with whom he was growing very serious. She was spending more and more time in his apartment, and that would necessarily infringe on some of the freedom he had previously had with me. He felt now, as he had felt two weeks earlier when he first told me this, that I was entitled to understand this new development in the situation.

"What did I say the first time you told me this?" I asked him sarcastically.

"You said that you would continue your relationship with me since I had not made an exclusive commitment to this other woman."

Five years later, I was to learn that he did, indeed, have this exact conversation. It was just as he had remembered it. But it had been with another patient!

There were also moments during and after our sexual encounters when it became difficult to discern if he was engaged in sexual fantasy, or if he had lost touch with reality. These moments occurred after our encounters had moved from masturbation to fellatio. He asked often, "See what you've been missing?" as if each time was my first. He might ask, "So, what do you think of sucking?" immediately following an episode of instructed fellatio. Or, "You never knew sex had so many variations, did you?" when the variation in our sex was negligible from one time to the next. This was disturbing to me not only because he knew from my disclosures in therapy that oral sex was not new to me, but predominantly because oral sex with him had been so frequent. Yet each time continued to be treated by him as if it were my first. "So what do you think of our little discovery?" I heard it often.

Signs of his confusion appeared in some of his instructions before sex, as well. Shortly after fellatio had become a regular routine for us, he became quite preoccupied with having me swallow his semen. The first time he told me to do this, he explained that healthy women can experience an orgasm at the moment the semen hit their palate. I had never had such an experience, but mine, I remembered, was an unfeminine past, not one from which to be drawing abstractions on psychological principles of mental health. I did not volunteer any contradictions to his knowledge.

Each time subsequent to that, when he would instruct me to "swallow it," he would always follow his order with the same story about female orgasms being evoked by the feeling of semen against the palate. Each time, he spoke as if there had been no time preceding it. Each time, he spoke as if this time was our first. Had he forgotten? Or was this a fantasy enactment: fellatio with a virgin? I did not know, nor did I question it. I knew that someday this would all become clear to me, someday when I was healthy.

His bizarre behavior only compounded the confusion I still experienced over our past and present. Still riddled with fear and guilt, I struggled to love him, to be perfectly healthy. And sometimes, when I was overwhelmed by the doubts and anxiety, I would question him on the nature of our relationship.

"We do not date, yet we do share a bed. We do not have intercourse, but I do fellate you. I do not take meals with you, yet I do take baths with you.

"This is not therapy. You told me so once. But I need to know—what is this?"

I never really expected to get an answer from him, and he never disappointed me.

The lack of understanding about what this all meant to Dr.

Leonard, what *I* meant to Dr. Leonard, grew progressively more frustrating and distressing. The lack of consistency and predictability confused me further. On which days would I be invited to his bedroom? Would he want to see me after this session? After this tape? Would he want me to spend the night? Would he not want to see me at all? Would that mean that I had done something to displease him?

Once, when I was leaving his bedroom, he said that next time he wanted me to ask if I could stay; he wanted it to be my idea. The following week, keeping in mind his request, I asked him if I could stay after the session. I looked to see approval in his eyes.

"No," he replied instead. "But don't let that keep you from asking again."

When the following week's videotape had ended, I waited for him in the living room. After his patient for that hour had left, I asked him if I could stay during his lunch hour.

"What for?" he asked playfully.

In the surprised silence that followed, I realized that I was really expected to answer.

"To play with you?" I answered in a questioning tone, as if to ask him if that was the right response.

After motioning me to follow him into the bedroom, he said that next time he wanted my answer to be more explicit. He didn't want me to say "play with" him. He wanted me to name exactly what I was going to be doing to him. Maybe because he always told me what to do *after* I got to his bedroom, I never was able to do that. And that disappointed him.

The most disturbing and hurtful behavior I witnessed during this time came just before the end of the summer. Again, he had asked me to be the one to initiate the next encounter, and so I asked if I could see him following my session. This time, he played no games. He agreed to see me, but added that he preferred it to be at the end of the day. I should, he told me, plan on spending the night.

He opened the door to me at our prearranged hour of eight-thirty. He was naked and holding a pencil. He asked me to go into the bedroom and wait for him; he had work to finish up in the office. I waited nearly an hour and a half before he joined me. This time he was holding a drink.

He sprawled out in the middle of the bed, still naked, still holding onto his glass. He was tired, but "nevertheless horny," he said. Could I do this quickly, he wondered. He wanted to go to sleep.

He told me what he wanted, and I performed as I always did. Within minutes, maybe less, it was over. He lay still for several moments and then he rose without a word. Carrying one of the pillows with him, he left the bedroom. When he returned, he was empty-handed.

"I want to sleep alone tonight," he said. "I've made a bed for you on the living room sofa."

I withdrew into myself, as I did so often when I was hurt beyond words. I said nothing, but walked dutifully into the living room. I carried my clothes with me, as he did not want to be disturbed in the morning before I left to catch the first train back to Yonkers.

"Why did you want me here tonight?" I asked him quietly.

"I didn't ask to see you. You asked to see me," he replied.

Aghast at this twisted interpretation of events, I momentarily accepted his remark and questioned why he had allowed me to invite myself.

"I didn't want to disappoint you," he answered.

He returned to his bed, and I was left standing in front of the living room window covered only by the darkness of his apartment around me. I watched the traffic of the cars and pedestrians below and listened to the noise that their commotion caused. And I felt my excruciating loneliness accentuated by the hustle and bustle of the streets. I wanted to go home. I wanted to hug my baby and sleep in my own bed. I wanted to sleep to the quiet sounds of the suburbs and leave the sirens and lights in a different world. I was twenty-one years old and I was aching with homesickness.

I cried until I knew I would be able to sleep. Then I looked at my watch and counted four hours before the first train to Yonkers would leave from Grand Central Station. I closed my eyes on the sofa that had been made a bed for me and vowed never to spend another night in that apartment. I never did.

There was no romantic or sexual satisfaction for me in my relationship with Dr. Leonard. It was not fulfilling for me in any way other than in the knowledge that he approved of me. I was not in love with him nor was I turned on by him. I was merely working toward the day when I would be and when the sign of my new mental health would make itself known. But there came a time, at the end of that summer, when my need to love and be loved became an emotional priority for me and a source of conflict with Dr. Leonard. I had found another man.

"My relationship with *Jack* is getting serious," I told him in a session. "I think I have fallen in love with him."

Jack was a friend from Chicago. When he was with a former girlfriend and I was with my former husband, we had double dated. Now we were seeing each other in a new light and finding that more than a friendship was there. Jack was also a patient of Dr. Leonard.

I went on to explain to Dr. Leonard that our bedroom relationship would obviously have to stop.

"What's so obvious about it?" he wanted to know. "Aren't you capable of loving two men simultaneously?" he asked as if I should be. "Aren't you feminine enough to show your love for two men?"

"But I would feel too guilty continuing this with you while pursuing a fuller relationship with Jack."

"Why should you feel guilty?" he asked with a bit of anger. "Have you broken a promise of exclusivity? Have you broken a commitment? What exactly do you think you're doing wrong?"

I had no answers that both felt and sounded as convincing as his rhetorical questions.

"Do you see any good reason why a woman cannot maintain more than one sexual relationship until she has a clear

84

understanding of which man is more worthy of her admiration?" he asked. "That is the only way she can make an informed decision," he told me.

I was being set up, and I knew it. It was clear that Dr. Leonard would have considered himself to be the more admirable of the two men. It was also clear that if that was *his* consideration, it should be mine, as well. Dr. Leonard was the healthy, moral, accomplished man; Jack was his patient and just starting out. Dr. Leonard was the living example of the perfect happiness to which we all aspired; Jack was still aspiring. The healthy woman was supposed to respond to the ideal man. I dared not say that I did not.

"What about the fact that you'd be having a sexual relationship with the girlfriend of a patient?" I asked.

"That is a matter strictly between that patient and me," he told me sternly. "If I didn't think I could remain objective in Jack's therapy, I would certainly terminate your relationship with me. But that is not the case, so I do not intend to consider the matter any further."

So our relationship continued as it had in the past. Morning and afternoon trips to the back of his apartment to rub his back and stimulate his penis continued for several more weeks until I felt myself disintegrating inside. I was, once again, being consumed with guilt.

I prepared myself for the session in which I would tell him that this had to end. I rehearsed how I would say that the first half of the year was still haunting me. It still created doubts and anxiety whenever I permitted myself to think about it, and I still had not been able to settle the questions I had. I would tell him that I knew that I would eventually come to understand those episodes if I continued to work hard in therapy. But this, this two men at the same time, this was something different.

I would explain to him that I felt like I was betraying Jack. Then I would tell him how much Jack meant to me and how I didn't want to jeopardize that relationship. I would tell him that I understood what Jack was offering me, what it was we had together; but what I had with Dr. Leonard, well, I didn't even know what that was.

I would tell him that I could not handle the guilt anymore. It was just that simple. Our situation, whatever it was, would have to end. That was all there was to it.

When I began that session for which I had so carefully rehearsed, the fear was written all over my face. Again, I was worn out from a sleepless night and numerous trips to the bathroom. But I told him what I had to say, albeit with much less firmness than I had felt during my last rehearsal in the privacy of my shower that morning, and he listened carefully.

"Do you feel you have chosen the better man?" he asked when I had finished.

He was baiting me again, and I was immediately intimidated.

"No, of course not." What other answer was possible? "It's just that Jack gives me the consistency and predictability that I need in a relationship, and you can't give me that."

He thought it over for a moment and then said, "Sometimes I guess it might be legitimate to choose context over quality."

With that, the issue was settled.

All of my therapy and all of my life was not fixated on my sexual relationship with Dr. Leonard. I tried to maintain as much normalcy as possible, and to a large extent succeeded. No one would have suspected what turmoil I suffered on the inside. I had easily learned to compartmentalize. It was this, I believe, that allowed me to function, to function well—and perhaps survive.

My personal life centered around making a life for my son and myself apart from my ex-husband. By August, I was able to afford the moving expenses involved in physically separating from David. My son Eric and I moved to a small apartment in Mt. Vernon, New York. For the first time, we were truly on our own. Up until that time, my separation had been signified by my sleeping on the floor of the baby's room or on the sofa bed in the living room that I ultimately bought for myself shortly before my move.

Caring for Eric filled my days. As a matter of fact, little else was included, which sometimes led to loneliness for adult conversation. I was the only one among my friends who had a child, and I was one of the few among my friends who did not live in Manhattan. So it was not so much by choice as it was by circumstance that Eric was often my sole company for days at a time.

I supposed that most parents felt as I did, but I really did believe that Eric was a remarkable child. He was not only the most beautiful child in the world, he was great fun to be with! We spent our hours together at the playground behind our apartment building, or walking to the nearby stores, or watching "Sesame Street," or reading storybooks. And sometimes, when it was time to lay him down for sleep, but I was not ready to be without him, I would just watch Eric in his crib and cry over the wonder of him. As I recall, it was, for the most part, a beautiful time for my baby and me.

My time with Eric was both fuel for my soul and escape from the other life I led—the life with Dr. Leonard. It was the place where judgments and condemnations did not exist, and giggles and hugs replaced considerations of right and wrong. He was what kept me grounded and centered. I am not sure whether it was because of how much I enjoyed him, or because I knew how much he needed me. I am only sure that he did.

My loneliness for adult company was somewhat relieved when Jack moved out of Manhattan to an apartment around the block from me in Mt. Vernon. We spent most of our evenings together, but the rockiness of our relationship told me that, as in love with Jack as I was, he would not be my permanent choice. I was still trying to break away from the role I had made for myself in marriage. I did not want to be someone else's cook, maid, and laundress. Jack, on the other hand, was never one inclined to carry out his share of household chores. He also had a penchant for being catered to. We were not a match made in heaven.

During this period, the relationship with my parents remained pretty stable. They even came out to visit me, once before I made the move to Mt. Vernon, and once after. And they had brought me out to Chicago on several occasions. But some things in the relationship with my mother never changed.

It was during this time that I received a telephone call from my mother telling me of her good news. "Your father and I are taking the whole family on a trip to Africa and Israel!" she announced.

"You're kidding," I answered stunned. I didn't know if there was going to be a punch line, or if indeed we were going on such an extravagant trip. I was not prepared for what was really going on.

"Your father and I have talked about this kind of trip for a long time," she was saying. She was mostly just rambling with excitment. "We thought it would be a wonderful trip to take our children on," she continued.

"When? When are we going?" I asked cautiously.

"Not you, Ellen," she answered. "Your brother and sister."

I couldn't speak. It was not, of course, that I would not see Africa and Israel with them that left me speechless. It was the ease with which Mommy could refer to her "whole family" or "our children" and not include me in those terms.

"Of course," I was finally able to respond. "How stupid of me," I thought.

"The trip isn't for a long time yet, but we'd love for you to see us off from Kennedy Airport," she added.

In the meantime, I continued to work on my therapy and at finding answers to so many long-standing questions. Whereas I would never discuss with anyone the encounters I had had with my doctor, I did find opportunities at social events to vent my doubts over Dr. Leonard's nude greetings at his front door. I never, of course, expressed the doubts themselves. Just the questions behind them.

"What do you think about that?" I might ask one of the women who had mentioned seeing Dr. Leonard in the buff. I searched her face for any clues that told me she felt the same uncertainty, nervousness, and concern that I was trying so hard not to feel and was so careful not to show. And I looked for signs that told me she had done more than just see him naked. With one exception, the women found his immodesty *beautiful*. Eventually, I convinced myself to see it the same way.

The one exception I encountered had served to demonstrate how severe my conflict indeed was. Having already questioned this particular woman on how she felt about his nudity in front of patients, I discovered that she was one of the few who not only had not been witness to this display, but did not know of its occurrence, either. As she became noticeably upset at this news, I found myself trying to soothe her with a defense of Dr. Leonard's behavior. The more upset she became, the more I tried to explain to her why he must be doing these nude prances through his apartment. My words fell on deaf ears, and she soon terminated her therapy. I felt guilty for years after about my role in her denying herself the best therapy that was available. Dr. Leonard diagnosed my guilt to be appropriate and well deserved.

But it wasn't until Dr. Leonard introduced nudity into my therapy sessions that the rumblings of a persistent conflict began to prepare for an eruption within me. He was working on an "innovative" therapy technique, he said, after he had finished reading *The Primal Scream*. Initially, he had just followed the techniques presented in this popular psychology book; he laid me on the floor in a spread-eagle position and worked with me toward derepressing.

Derepression, he explained, is the process of experiencing and remembering an event or a feeling that has been blocked out of consciousness, usually, but not always, because of pain associated with that event or feeling at the time it first occurred. Dr. Leonard, with the techniques he learned from *The Primal Scream* and his own questions, would lead the patient from the present time to a time in the past, a time which held a signifi-cant event or emotion for the patient. Together, they would work on getting that patient to experience that blocked memory.

It was not unusual to begin a session with Dr. Leonard in-structing me to lie on the floor so that we could "explore emo-tions." He would adjust the video camera to focus on the floor where I lay and he would come from behind his desk and sit on the floor a few feet away. Then, not unlike a hypnotist, he would take me back to when I was sixteen years old, thirteen years old, eleven, ten, eight. . . .

"Now call to your daddy," he would instruct. Or, "Tell your mother how you feel when she hits you." Thus would begin our hour of exploration.

Occasionally, but not often, these sessions were effective. There was much in my past that needed to be uncovered, and as I searched for these experiences or cried in response to their discovery, Dr. Leonard would sometimes hold me. Gently, pa-ternally, soothingly, he would rock me in his arms in a way that told me that no harm could come to me here. I relished these moments of safety and security. Whereas they painfully re-minded me of a time when I had ached for such reassurance, they also provided me the opportunity to fulfill that need now. And they assured me of Dr. Leonard's concern with my well-being. These hours told me that he had only my best interest at heart, that he would never do me harm, that he cared about me.

Soon after he ventured into this new avenue of psycho-therapy, however, he introduced his own new technique which, he claimed, was designed to quicken the derepression process.

It was in the late autumn when I arrived for this particular session. I took the patient's chair in his office and watched while he set the camera in place and the tape machine in operation. He took his seat behind the desk and asked me to remove my clothes—"all of them."

"What?" I asked him.

"Take off your clothes," he instructed. "I want to try a new technique. I think it will help you derepress faster."

I rose. I did not strip. I could feel my blood rushing through my hands and fingers. My head was spinning and my breathing had, all of a sudden, become very difficult. I sat down again.

"I can't do that," I told him.

He remained calm, much to my surprise. "I want you to trust me," he said. "Do you trust me?"

"Yes."

"I want you to be open with me," he said. "Do you want to be?"

I did not respond.

"Would it be easier if I did it for you?" he asked.

I did not question the alternatives nor his right to limit them so. Strip or be stripped. I could not bring myself to do it, so I chose the second alternative.

With the camera still rolling, he moved toward me and came around to the back of my chair. He untucked my blouse from behind me and slipped it over my head and arms. Then he unsnapped my bra and placed it over my blouse on the floor.

He moved in front of me and, taking my hands, signaled me to stand. When he placed his hands on the elastic of my skirt waist, I told him that I would finish it myself.

I stood naked in front of my therapist and his camera. I felt powerless and humiliated, and ashamed for feeling so. After all, did I not trust this man?

He motioned me to lie down and he began asking his questions, trying to guide me backwards in time. I tried to concentrate on what he was asking me, but I could only be aware of his and his camera's eye on my body. Nothing was accomplished that hour, but he seemed proud of me, nonetheless.

In future derepression sessions he would refuse to begin until all of my clothes had been removed. Often, that took more than half of my hour with him.

"I can't," I would tell him.

"Won't," he would return.

"*Can't.* I can't take my clothes off," I would insist.

"*Won't* take your clothes off," he would argue.

"I want to do whatever you think is best for me, but I just can't do *this.*"

"Won't," he repeated.

"It feels like *can't!*" I protested.

He urged me to force my way through those irrational fears that were preventing me from doing what I knew was right. If he persisted patiently and gently, then I felt guilty over being such a difficult patient for him. If he persisted with frustration and anger, I felt intimidated and scared. Either way, I ended up naked.

I never knew when these naked sessions would occur. Would this session be for derepressing, or would it be a lecture? The uncertainty only added to my nervousness beforehand. The sessions themselves served as a constant reminder of a past that would not die; the questions and doubts I had tried to ignore for so many months were now overwhelming my therapy—and my life.

It was in November of 1972 that I first heard about standards for professional behavior set by medical and psychiatric organizations. That was when I first learned that sexual relations between a therapist and his patient were considered to be a breach of the professional ethics set forth by the American Psychiatric Association. This information proved to be a turning point in my relationship with Dr. Leonard.

I had never before considered the sexual activity between Dr. Leonard and me as an issue of professional indiscretion or a violation of ethical standards. Now that I had heard that there was such a stand on this matter by members of his profession and that this stand denounced such activity, I began, for the first time, to doubt Dr. Leonard.

I wondered whether my inability to handle that first night in his bed was really a sign of my poor mental health. I wondered if my inability to climax at his ejaculations into my mouth was indeed a sign of diminished femininity. I wondered if my resistance and reluctance had really been signs of neurosis. I wondered about it all.

And then I wondered whether it was possible that the brilliant Dr. Leonard had done something wrong. Could it be that he had made a mistake? Could it be that this was all due to his ignorance over the professional standards for his field? Or was I looking for a scapegoat for my own inability to deal with the turmoil our relationship had caused me?

If he was right in any of what he had done, then, I thought, my continuing turmoil was a conclusive sign of basic instability and neurosis. On the other hand, there was this remote possibility that this was *his* problem, *his* error, *his* misjudgment. And if it was, I would have to terminate therapy with him. I would want to. He had gone to such an extreme with me, that there could be no going back.

I needed to understand. Who was at fault here? Was it me in my neurosis, or him in his judgment? I knew I was too involved, too emotional, and too confused to reach an understanding on the matter. I needed help. The only person to whom I had always turned for help had consistently denied me dialogue on this particular issue. Besides, now Dr. Leonard could not be trusted to have the requisite knowledge or objectivity. I would, I decided, call Dr. Blumenthal.

I think Dr. Blumenthal recognized my name when I phoned him, but I still reminded him of our conversation a year and a half earlier when he had recommended Dr. Leonard to me. He said he remembered it. I told him that I had followed his recommendation and had sought therapy from Dr. Leonard.

"Why, then," he wanted to know, "are you calling me?"

"Because I don't know if I should stay in therapy with Dr. Leonard," I replied.

Before I could continue, he interrupted. "I can't talk to you about this while you're still Dr. Leonard's patient."

"You don't understand," I explained. "There are circumstances that make it impossible for me to discuss this dilemma with Dr. Leonard. I used to try, but Dr. Leonard won't discus it, and now I need to talk to someone else about it."

"Please don't say any more. It would not be proper for me to assist you while you are under another doctor's care."

I continued anyway. "*Something* is going on between my therapist and me, and I just want you to tell me if that *something* is appropriate. If it is appropriate, I'll have no cause for leaving Dr. Leonard. In that case, I'd want to stay and work through my problems. But if it isn't appropriate, I'll leave therapy. I just need to know if what he is doing is or isn't right."

I was about to explain what the *something* was when he interrupted me. "I know what you're talking about, Ellen. I just can't help you."

"No, I don't think you can know what I am talking about, Dr. Blumenthal. What I am trying to say is . . ."

"I know *exactly* what you're talking about, Ellen, and I do not want you to say any more about it. If you would like to call me after you have terminated therapy with Dr. Leonard, I will speak to you then."

"But I don't want to terminate if he hasn't done anything wrong. If it's my problem, I should stay with Dr. Leonard and work it through. So I need to know if it's me or if it's him." I was hoping for a sign, a clue, as to what he thought.

"I'm sorry. That's all I can say. Good-bye." And he hung up.

"Damn you," I said into the dead receiver.

I had a date with Jack that night, but my mind was not with him. I was preoccupied and depressed, and it showed.

"Jack," I plunged right in, "do you think it's okay for a doctor to have sexual contact with a patient?"

He went white. It was the surprise at a question that had come out of nowhere, and the realization of what the question meant, all at once. His gazed disbelief told me I had asked the wrong person.

He barraged me with questions. He wanted to know so many things. And I, in my panic over the Pandora's box I had opened, would not so much as acknowledge his first question: "Why are you asking, Ellen?"

He knew, but I could not confirm what he thought he knew. He grew progressively more disturbed over the prospect of what he was thinking and pressed me for answers. I continued to refuse to answer.

"If you won't answer my questions, then maybe Dr. Leonard will," he said in frustration.

"No!" I begged him. "Please don't even tell him that you suspect anything." I was panicky. I felt a need to protect and defend Dr. Leonard from the judgment I read in Jack's eyes, and a need to protect myself from the fury that I knew would come from Dr. Leonard.

It was too late. The damage had been done.

"I'm sorry, Ellen," he told me, "but I don't know if I can continue with my therapy unless Dr. Leonard can either deny or explain the conclusion I have in my mind right now." He would, he said, have to speak with Dr. Leonard about this in his next session.

December 5, 1972

My session fell a week before Jack's. I was grateful for that bit of luck, as I thought it would be better if I told Dr. Leonard what happened myself, rather than have Jack walk into his session and spring this on an unprepared Dr. Leonard.

By now I had forgotten the events that had led up to my questioning of Jack in the first place. I had forgotten about the decision I was trying to make and the dilemma I had experienced. I had forgotten about professional ethics and doubts over his behavior. I was feeling only guilt and fear: guilt over having betrayed Dr. Leonard and fear over the consequences for having done so.

"I have an apology to make to you," I began the session. Then I told him about my evening with Jack.

He was reclining in his chair with his feet on his desk. With the folder pressed up against his lap, he had begun to write in my file when I first began to speak. Now he was slowly placing the folder and his pen on the desk.

"Go on," he said solemnly.

I explained, as best I could, what had led up to the question I had asked Jack. "You know how confused and upset I was after that first night in your bed. I just got more and more upset about it each time I thought about it and each time you would refuse to discuss it or answer my questions.

"Lately, it was so bad that I even considered the possibility that you had done something unethical with me." Then I told him what I had learned about the APA and its ethical standards. "But of course now I understand how severe my problems must have been to have had such reactions." He interrupted me here.

"Did you tell anyone else? Anyone? I want the names of everyone you have mentioned this to."

I looked away from his searching stare. I dreaded what was coming, but I knew it had to be told.

"Dr. Blumenthal. I sort of told Dr. Blumenthal. I didn't discuss anything with him, but I tried to. He wouldn't let me."

"Tell me what you said. Tell me everything you said and everything he said." He was delivering a dulled monotone order. It was controlled rage I was hearing.

I told him about my conversation with Dr. Blumenthal. He kept demanding more detail. "What did you say?" was followed by, "And what did he say?" which was followed again by, "And what did you say then?" which was sometimes followed by, "Is that *exactly* what you said?"

I answered his questions, and then went on to explain how that had led into my evening with Jack. When I was finished, there was a terrible silence.

He still had not moved or changed positions since having replaced his pen and folder on the desk. He still stared at me, but not with the bug eyes I had come to expect when he got angry. He almost looked as if he had not been listening to me. Looking at me, yes; listening to me, no.

Then he slowly brought his feet to the floor and swiveled the chair to face center. He leaned over his desk and quietly asked, "And you've told no one else?"

"No one," I replied.

"Just Jack and Dr. Blumenthal?" he verified.

"Just Jack and Dr. Blumenthal."

There was more silence. Now his eyes began to bulge as they slowly filled with rage. Then he broke the silence.

"You're scum," I heard him say. "You're real scum."

My probation session had begun. I had already been scared and ashamed before my therapist called me "scum," judged my womanhood to be so far less than what he had previously thought, and promised never to touch me again. I had hoped to find forgiveness and relief from my guilt in his office. Instead, I found only a growing sense of worthlessness. In less than an hour, I would begin my contemplation of the alternate methods available for killing myself.

9

A◇MERRY
CHRISTMAS

Just before the commencement of my next scheduled visit, Dr. Leonard entered a note to himself in my record. Written just beneath the stamped imprint of that day's date was:

Plan: Continue business as usual.

And so he did. He did not refer to that previous session, not during that hour nor during any of the hours that ever followed. Taking my cue from my doctor, I did not mention it either, not until four years later.

Though we each acted as if that probationary session had never occurred, it was, nevertheless, ever present in the therapy that followed. It dictated my unquestioning obedience, my further suppression of confusion over past sexual encounters, and my fervor to regain my therapist's favor. And it left me feeling that I had only two options: to give up my life, or to give my life to him. I chose the latter.

With my return to that December 19 session, the gradual suspension of my judgment, of my values, and of my own sense of self, which had begun so early in my therapy, was all but complete. My life was now totally his to mold, alter, and judge however he saw fit.

He continued to give and I continued to follow old orders, and he found new ones to levy, as well. It was not a conscious decision that motivated my obedience, nor did I bring to conscious memory any detailed rerun of that probationary session before following his commands. I simply obeyed. Whatever choice I may have had to obey or not, had been subsumed and irrevocably decided with the act of resuming therapy and "business as usual." My obedience was automatic. To have evaluated his words was not an option I considered open, much less to have disobeyed them. It would have been like questioning the rightness of breathing; as it is an automatic process for survival, so I experienced my obedience to my therapist. Without doubt, without guilt, without thought, I performed with conviction and belief the role he set out to prescribe for me. And the better I performed, the more positive his response, the greater my sense of self-worth.

I felt no resistance to surrendering my identity to this man. On the contrary, I was eager to behave in any manner he desired in order to regain his faith, and I looked for any opportunity to do so. I did not struggle to maintain my own sense of judgment; I suspended it, substituting his for mine. I did not question his lectures on a morality that felt alien to mine; I incorporated his code as my own. I did not doubt his advice on healthier and happier living; I worked earnestly to integrate his ideas into my behavior. I did not challenge his evaluations of me; I translated his evaluations into my own self-esteem. If he liked me, I liked myself. If he disapproved of me, I felt lost and abandoned. It seemed a matter of life and death that he like me; he was my lifeline and without him I could not survive.

Ours was not unlike the relationship between an abusive parent and an abused child. I learned to read his face, his movements, and his tone of voice with precision and accuracy. Always careful not to displease him, I needed to see his storms brewing before they became too strong to dissipate. I cautiously balanced disclosures that might prove how much I trusted him with those I felt might anger him. I monitored the manner in which I spoke to him, as constant admiration and respect seemed to evoke gentler handling of me in sessions. I defended him at any hint of attack or disapproval by another, even when such an attack had long since passed and he was relaying the incident to me himself. And I feared him to the point of physical illness before each visit to his office, as much as I sought him out for love and acceptance.

One of the old orders that remained unchanged was his requirement that I remove my clothes for many of my sessions. Whereas the hesitation and nervousness persisted, I was always quick to inform him that I knew my modesty in front of him was still a problem and that I was working harder than ever on correcting it. And I was.

"I'm trying," I told him when I felt too much time had elapsed between his command to strip and my standing up to do so. "I know this should be easy for me, but it isn't."

"Just make yourself do it," he would order. "Force your way through those irrational feelings that are keeping you from doing what you know is best." Then he would tell me the story of the hypothetical patient who had a doorknob phobia.

"If a patient came to me with a fear of doorknobs, how would you suggest I treat him?"

Certain that he intended to answer the question for me, I said nothing.

"If such a patient came to me, I would make him touch as many doorknobs as I could find for him. I would make him force his way through those fears, for only in doing so will he come to learn that no harm comes from touching doorknobs."

Whenever he posed that question to me, no answer was needed. Its function was not to invite dialogue, but to make me disrobe.

I made remarkable *progress* during those months in therapy. Somewhere I remembered that, should I not progress faster than all his other patients, I would be expelled. I continued, without exception, to perform in accordance with all the rules set for my probation. And he seemed genuinely pleased with our work.

"You know," he said again as I departed from one of my sessions, "you could not get this kind of help anywhere else."

"Yes, I know," I responded with admiration.

"Do you want to say something to me?" he suggested.

"I want to thank you for keeping me as a patient." I thought that was what I was supposed to say.

"Is that all?" he asked.

I had read him incorrectly, but now I knew for sure what was expected. "No," I continued, "I want to tell you I love you, too."

He smiled. "Doesn't it feel better to say it and get it out, than to keep it bottled up inside?"

I smiled back in agreement, and left.

These months of therapy turned into a year, but as obedient as I had been that year, no mention was made of my probation being terminated. I did not dare ask what my status was, as it was understood by its obvious omission from conversations that the subject, like that of sex between him and me, was off-limits. So my therapy continued in much the same manner, as I knew I had even more to prove to my therapist.

My personal life during these years proceeded as it had before. More adept than ever at keeping the events surrounding my therapist separate from the rest of my life, my activities and relationships showed no visible signs of alteration as a result of past events.

My relationship with Jack continued only for a few months past my probation session, but it did so as if nothing had happened. Apparently satisfied with whatever explanation Dr. Leonard had given, Jack continued his therapy without interruption, and we never discussed the matter again.

Sometime after Jack and I had agreed that the time had passed for each of us to seek elsewhere a higher percentage of what we were needing, I moved into the city. This brought me closer to my friends and relieved the growing sense of isolation I had felt in the suburbs.

I became involved with *Jonathan*, another of Dr. Leonard's patients. This affair deepened and progressed for some time.

But my son continued to be the center of my life. Motherhood and the relationship with Eric were an ever increasing source of satisfaction and pleasure with each year of his growth. It provided me with not only an outlet for deeply felt love and attachment, but with a certain continuity and stability, as well. For a life otherwise devoid of such necessities, these were critical. And as it had been most clearly the existence of that little person, so full of love and life, that had kept me from killing myself the night of my probationary session, it was also that child who brought freshness and energy to each day since.

I enrolled Eric in a Montessori school only eight blocks from where we lived, hired a full-time babysitter to take him to and pick him up from the half-day program, and went to work for the first time since having my child. It bothered me that I would not be home for him when he returned from school each day and that we wouldn't have the afternoons to be together. But money was very tight and I knew it was time to start earning my own way. Child support would not last forever, and for sure it was inadequate.

It was sometime in the middle of 1974 when the full extent of my *progress* in therapy became apparent to me. Recalling the numerous times Dr. Leonard had asked me if I trusted him and had asked me to prove it, I thought to myself, with deep satisfaction, that I did trust him completely. I fantasized in a deep daydream that he was asking that same question of me now: "Do you trust me, Ellen?" When I tell him that I do, he asks if I would do anything he asked me to do in order to prove it. I tell him that I would. Then he asks me to jump off the Empire State Building, promising at the same time that no harm will come to me. "Just trust me," he says in my fantasy.

I agree to this demonstration of trust and he leads me by the hand to the rooftop of the skyscraper. I move to the ledge, and as I prepare to position myself for the jump, I look back at him for reassurance. He smiles at me and, once again, says, "Trust me." I turn around to face the sky and my mission. And I jump.

This fantasy did not alarm me. On the contrary, it showed me how far I had progressed in my therapy from the days of questioning his behavior in light of the APA's code of ethics. It showed me that I was capable of trust in and reliance on Dr. Leonard, a phenomenon he said he considered essential to beneficial therapy.

I spent much time in fantasy during those middle years of therapy, and one in particular predominated. I see myself in a courtroom, on the witness stand. Dr. Leonard is being tried for sexually molesting his female patients which, in my fantasy, is a criminal offense. If convicted, he will go to prison for life.

Women have already testified prior to my appearance about what Dr. Leonard has done to them, and it looks certain that he will be convicted. But now it is my turn to speak.

Before any question is put to me, I announce to the court that the trial of this great man is a travesty. There is no way, I tell them, that they could possibly understand the workings of this genius nor appreciate the complexity of what he is trying to accomplish. I tell them that it is their own sexual repression that causes them to judge his greatness as a crime.

Then noticing that the judge is a woman, I tell Her Honor that her mere presence on the bench in this trial is clear proof that she lacks femininity, because a healthy woman would have the ability to see the injustice being done here, and, accordingly, step down. I close my remarks with a general statement on the unhealthy psychologies of all those who are accusing and attempting to judge him.

My speech is so stirring that, of course, he is acquitted, And he, knowing who it is that is responsible for his freedom, is forever indebted to me.

I never interpreted these fantasies as an indication that our sexual encounters were still a source of unresolved turmoil. I saw them, instead, as symbolic of the forward movement I had made in my therapy. I was getting better.

Dr. Leonard thought I was getting better, too. He not only said this in some of my sessions, but his actions out of therapy confirmed the diagnosis. Once, for example, I invited him to a party I was giving. Much to my surprise, he accepted the invitation. Questioning whether the acceptance was motivated from a lack of something better to do with his evening or from a genuine wish to share my company, I extended a second invitation to another gathering not too long after the first. He accepted that one, as well. Now I felt honored.

On a different occasion, he invited me to join him for dinner at the neighborhood coffee shop following my session at the end of the day. I was elated. I might still be on probation, I thought, but I am clearly special to this man.

It was at the end of 1974, two years following my probation session, when Dr. Leonard bestowed the ultimate compliment on me. He invited me to his home for a Christmas party.

Fifteen *select* patients had been invited to this party. Honored to have been so, each one was certain to attend. Jonathan and I arrived shortly after the others and were invited to place our coats in the master bedroom and help ourselves to a drink from the kitchen.

Liquor, mixers, and glasses cluttered the limited counter space. I ignored the wines and hard drinks, and poured myself a soda before returning to the tree decorating festivities in the living room. The focus, however, was less centered on the tree than it was on Dr. Leonard.

As the evening wore on and the tree was completed, the entertainment took a new form. Dr. Leonard's girlfriend, Patricia Street, led us in song, along with her guitar-playing accompanist and friend. We sang together, we listened to Pat and her partner sing alone, and we laughed at Dr. Leonard's attempts to carry a solo or drown out the chorus. Everyone seemed to be truly enjoying themselves.

It was when the guitarist needed to rest his fingers that I seized an opportunity to refill my drink. I was alone in the kitchen when I was startled by Dr. Leonard's presence.

"Give me a kiss," he said, while grabbing me from behind.

I whirled around, throwing him off balance, and proclaimed, "You scared me!" I pushed him away as I spoke.

"Just one kiss," he pleaded coyly.

Again, I had to push him away. "Pat's probably waiting for you in the living room. She'll be wondering what happened to you."

"Just one," he insisted, "then I'll leave you alone."

With that, he pushed me against the dishwasher and moved his face toward mine.

"No!" I stated firmly, and I pushed him aside.

I did not understand what he was doing. He had sworn during my probation session that he would never touch me again.

I dismissed the possibility of finding an answer, and quickly moved into the living room to find Jonathan. When I found him, I did not mention Dr. Leonard's behavior in the kitchen. I just joined him on the living room rug where he was seated and started a private conversation.

"May I join you?" I heard Dr. Leonard ask from behind us. I turned around to see he was addressing the question to my date.

Dr. Leonard took the spot on the right side of me while my date remained fixed at my left.

"Do you like to get tickled?" Dr. Leonard asked in a threatening tone.

"I hate it," I replied sternly, looking right into his eyes.

"How about this? Does this tickle?" he asked as he poked his finger into my ribs.

"Don't," I warned.

"*Don't?* Did you say *don't?*"

With that, he pushed my shoulders down to the floor, throwing my body back. He quickly moved in the opposite direction where my legs were extended in front of me. He grabbed my ankles tightly, and pressed my legs hard against the ground.

"Get her shoulders!" he called to Jonathan. "Kneel on her shoulders!"

Jonathan did not hesitate. Before I was able to pull my torso all the way up, he was pulling me down again.

I had never liked this kind of playing, not even as a child. I liked it even less now. Being trapped or overpowered always scared me, and I was scared now.

"Please, Jonathan," I begged, looking directly at him, "please don't do this."

Not seeing that I was serious, Jonathan continued in Dr. Leonard's game. I pleaded again, this time holding back the tears that were ready to flow.

"Jonathan, I mean it. Stop!"

Sensing the seriousness of my discomfort this time, he released me immediately and later apologized. Dr. Leonard followed suit in releasing me, but called us "poor sports" and left.

Jonathan and I stood, and decided not to sit again until sofa or chair space opened up. Dr. Leonard moved on to other guests, joking with some of the men and dancing to no music with some of the women. Then he took a seat on the floor next to one of his male patients.

"Tony," Dr. Leonard said, "who's got the better boxing team? Navy or Marines?" It wasn't a serious question the former naval officer was posing to this ex-Marine. He was having fun.

"Let's hear it for the Marines!" Tony cheered in reply.

"Oh yeah?" Dr. Leonard teased back. With that, he pounced on Tony to feign a match of their own. "Who's got the best team?"

"The Marines!" his patient cheered on, this time with laughter.

Dr. Leonard pinned Tony to the floor and persisted in the roughhousing he had started. "What?" he questioned playfully.

This time Tony did not need to reply, for his demonstration of superior strength in escaping Dr. Leonard's grip made all the statement for the Marines that was needed. He laughed at his victory, and at the fun he was having with the man whom he loved so much.

Dr. Leonard lunged toward Tony to reestablish his position, but Tony was too swift for the doctor. It was Tony who ended up in control of Dr. Leonard. Now, with a different expression on his face, Dr. Leonard jerked his knee upward in aim of

106

Tony's testicles. Only Dr. Leonard's lack of leverage spared Tony the intended pain.

Tony saw that viciousness had replaced humor on Dr. Leonard's face, and looking into his therapist's eyes, Tony suggested that they "cool it."

"That's enough," Tony declared, and he released his grip on the weaker man.

"You shouldn't have done that," Dr. Leonard said coldly.

"Shouldn't have done what?" Tony asked.

"You shouldn't have done that," he repeated.

With that, Dr. Leonard threw a punch that caused blood to run from his patient's lip. The room fell silent and all eyes turned to the two men.

"What the hell . . . ?" Tony was stunned and confused as he fought to hold back the tears.

"Go on, hit me!" the doctor goaded.

"I don't want to hit you, Dr. Leonard," Tony replied with bewilderment.

Dr. Leonard grimaced and then he struck Tony again.

"*Now* hit me back," he taunted.

"I don't want to fight with you. I love you." Tony was beginning to lose the struggle against his tears.

Fury paralyzed Dr. Leonard's bug eyes into a glare that forewarned what was to follow. Tony made a move to escape, but the doctor had him trapped. Tony's only alternative to what he saw coming was to strike his beloved therapist and he gave no indication that he considered the alternative viable. He would have won such an altercation, and that, he would explain some time later, is part of what stopped him.

"Come on, hit me!" Dr. Leonard ordered again. Then he charged his guest with the ferociousness of a wild animal. He struck Tony in the face again and again, each punch rendering Tony more helpless. When he could swing no more, his arms fell limp by his sides and he taunted once again, "Come and get me!"

Tony found his way to his feet and staggered off the living

room rug into the dining area. Tears ran down his face, blending with the blood that poured from his wounds.

"Why are you doing this?" he begged of his doctor. "What do you want?"

"Come on, Tony. Come and get me," Dr. Leonard continued. He was still taunting Tony and there was no sign that the violence had ended.

When Tony did not move toward Dr. Leonard, Dr. Leonard moved toward Tony, this time grabbing him by the shirt and dragging him into the kitchen. Though we heard the sound of breaking glass, no one made a move to investigate the cause. Only I was crying, and only I spoke.

"Can't you do anything to make him stop?" I asked Dr. Leonard's girlfriend, Patricia.

Sitting on the floor, calmly leaning back on the palms of her hands, Pat casually replied, "He knows what he's doing. Don't worry about it."

My lord, I thought, is this some kind of therapy? I quickly remembered the last time I had asked that question, and I chose to remain silent now.

Moments after they had entered the kitchen, Tony came stumbling out, as if he had been thrown. Dr. Leonard followed, and opened the closet door adjacent to the kitchen. He reached up to the shelf above the hanging rack and pulled out a gun.

Tony was barely able to stand as the awareness of the weapon registered in his eyes. Covered with blood, toothless, and dazed, he was nevertheless conscious enough to perceive this new threat.

"Take it," Dr. Leonard ordered. "Take the gun from me."

I thought the order was a dare.

"Put the gun away, Dr. Leonard. *Please* put it away." Tony was begging for us all.

"I said take the gun, damn it!" he screamed, as he rammed the gun into Tony's hands. Then he stood back a foot or so and issued his next command.

"Shoot me!" he ordered. "Go on, shoot me. You've got the gun. Use it. I can't stop you. Shoot!"

Tony quickly looked for someone who would risk standing up to take the gun from him. Someone did, and the gun was whisked away to the back of the apartment.

Dr. Leonard barged toward the front door and threw it open. "Get out!" he screamed to Tony. "Get the hell out of here!"

Tony refused to leave. "I want an explanation," Tony demanded in between the sobs. "I'm not leaving until I get an explanation."

"You're violating my property rights!" Dr. Leonard accused. The Objectivist psychotherapist was accusing his patient of the equivalent of a mortal sin in Objectivism. "You say you love me and then you violate my property rights? You don't love me if you can do that. You don't love me at all."

He moved toward Tony again, this time grabbing him by the collar and back of his shirt, and threw him out of his apartment into the outer hallway. Now the rest of us were rising to retrieve our coats and leave this Christmas party.

We found Tony on the floor of the hall when we emerged from the apartment. Dazed and crying, he would tell me later that, in that moment, he felt he was having a nervous breakdown. I did not think about what I should do. I just knelt down beside Tony and held him. We were mere acquaintances before this evening, but now I felt that we were soul twins.

When he was ready, I helped him off the floor and walked him slowly to my apartment. I was the party guest who lived closest to Dr. Leonard; it made sense that Tony come home with me. We were joined by several others whose concern for Tony and need to talk led to a late night vigil.

I cleaned Tony's face, listened to him while he rambled in a state of confusion, and stroked his head to calm him until he was ready to sleep. That night was the beginning of the most important friendship I had ever had.

Once Tony had fallen asleep in my bedroom, the rest of us talked in the living room about what we had witnessed that evening. We hypothesized on what possible explanation there could be for that night's crisis, as we looked for reason where there was none. No one knew exactly what we should do, so we waited.

Early in the morning, shortly after sunrise, and after most of the crowd had gone home to sleep, my telephone rang.

"Ellen, this is Dr. Leonard. Is Tony there?"

"He is, but he's sleeping."

We both spoke calmly and without emotion.

"Would you please wake him up?" he requested.

"No, I won't. He needs to sleep."

"Would you tell him I'm on the phone and ask him if he'd like to get up?" he asked.

"No, Dr. Leonard. I don't think he should be disturbed."

He accepted my refusal without further discussion. He asked me to tell Tony to expect a call later in the day. Then he explained that he would later be calling the other guests who had witnessed last night's melée, after he had had a chance to speak with Tony.

"I'll wait for your call," I replied. "Good-bye."

"Good-bye."

When Tony awoke, it was late in the morning. I relayed Dr. Leonard's message, and Tony and I talked about what he could expect from the coming conversation with his doctor. When we had exhausted all the possibilities we could imagine, Tony left for home, a shower, clean clothes, and to await Dr. Leonard's phone call. I resolved to stay in my apartment where I could wait to hear from my new friend when he had finished talking to Dr. Leonard, and from Dr. Leonard himself.

Tony and Dr. Leonard arranged to meet at one o'clock that same afternoon. The discussion was set at Tony's convenience, as Dr. Leonard seemed most eager to accommodate him. The meeting place was to be Dr. Leonard's office.

Before he began, Dr. Leonard put his video machine into operation, and turned the camera on himself. He wanted, he explained, to see his face when he said the things he was about to say to Tony.

Dr. Leonard began his explanation of what had transpired

the night before. He had been drunk, he said, so drunk that he lost control of himself. He did, however, remember what had provoked him to hit Tony. It was, he claimed, his "subconscious calling out for justice."

Tony did not grasp the meaning of Dr. Leonard's explanation, so Dr. Leonard had to clarify the point. He explained that when he had first tried to hurt Tony with his knee, Tony should have retaliated. When Tony did not, but released Dr. Leonard instead, Dr. Leonard became enraged at the injustice Tony had allowed. With each punch that followed, Dr. Leonard said he was trying to provoke Tony into a *just* retaliation. Tony's refusal to defend himself or punish Dr. Leonard only served to fuel the therapist's rage. Now his explanation was being understood by Tony. At least, the words were.

At this point, Tony questioned his doctor on the cruelty and hostility that had accompanied this plea for justice from Dr. Leonard's subconscious. That was not hostility, Dr. Leonard told him. That was, the therapist analyzed, Tony's own projection of Tony's father onto Dr. Leonard, the therapist. It was a common phenomenon, he assured Tony. "It's called *transference.*"

Transference, he explained, is the occurrence wherein a patient *transfers* the feelings he has about one of his parents onto the therapist, or *transfers* the image of one of his parents onto the therapist. The parent involved in this transference of feeling or perception is usually the parent with whom the patient had the most difficulty. In this case, it was clear to Dr. Leonard that Tony, an abused child, had seen his father's face in Dr. Leonard. It was not viciousness from Dr. Leonard which Tony had witnessed, it was the viciousness he had seen all too often coming from his father.

With an unsettling discomfort, Tony, for the moment, accepted the doctor's analysis, as well as his denial of cruelty. Dr. Leonard continued on to his next point.

Reparation, he explained, is a major part of justice. He had injured Tony last night, and was now asking what payment Tony wanted for the harm he had caused.

Tony knew that major dental work would be required to repair the damage that Dr. Leonard had done and payment for that repair work was all that he sought. Dr. Leonard agreed to Tony's request and promised to set him up with his own dentist.

Dr. Leonard then proceeded to his fourth and last point. Dr. Leonard was issuing himself, he told Tony, a self-imposed punishment, one which he felt was in proportion to his offense: he would never drink alcohol again. Never. Not for the rest of his life. He would make the same announcement to us all before the weekend ended. He would announce the revocation of his punishment less than two years later.

When their conversation had ended, Dr. Leonard invited Tony to join him and Pat in the living room. There they spent the next three hours discussing sports and economics, and drinking coffee together. They treated Tony like an old friend, as they all attempted to put behind them a night that should never have happened.

Before Tony left Dr. Leonard's apartment, Dr. Leonard telephoned me to set up a time for our discussion. We agreed upon seven o'clock, but at my place, not his, much to his annoyance. I could not see myself scurrying to find a babysitter at this late hour, much less paying for one, and I told him so.

"Jonathan is with me now," I told him, "so you needn't call him, too. He'll be here tonight when you arrive."

"And I'll bring Pat along—for a witness," he replied.

Tony walked from Dr. Leonard's apartment to mine. He appeared more relaxed than the last time I had seen him and actually managed a smile when I greeted him. He took a seat at the dining room table where Jonathan and I had been talking. I resumed my place and waited for Tony to speak.

"I'm satisfied," he told us. He said nothing more.

"What happened?" I asked, confused by his brevity.

"That's all I'm at liberty to say," Tony explained. Dr. Leonard had extracted a promise from Tony to keep their conversation confidential. All that Tony was free to relay was his acceptance of Dr. Leonard's explanation and reparation. It was not until years later that the content of that meeting between Tony and Dr. Leonard was ever revealed to me. Up until 1977, this was a well-kept secret between this patient and his doctor. Had the explanation been revealed to me at the time Tony received it, I doubt my acceptance would have been any different from Tony's. As bizarre and unsettling as Dr. Leonard's explanation was, I still would have given him the benefit of my own self-doubt.

My doorbell rang promptly at seven. As Dr. Leonard and Pat walked in, Tony rose to leave, exchanging amenities with Dr. Leonard on his way out. Dr. Leonard sat where Tony had just been, and Pat to his left. Jonathan and I sat next to one another, across from them at the table. Then Dr. Leonard spoke.

"The major issue," Dr. Leonard said, "is between Tony and me." He said that he recognized the discomfort we may have experienced over his behavior, but reminded us that the damage had been done to Tony, not us.

"I fixed it with Tony, and you can verify that fact with Tony. But the details of that are private between Tony and me."

"That's it?" I asked. "That's all the explanation we get?"

"Well, yes, other than expressing my hope that you won't let this interfere with your treatment. I see no reason, though, why it should.

"If you judge the full context of everything you know about me and my overall character, I think you'll find that the benefit I am to you far outweighs whatever I did last night. And since you were not the injured party, there really is nothing more to say than that."

I could not believe that we would not get *any* explanation. Would this, too, remain an unanswered mystery? I was almost frantic for some sort of statement on the matter of his behavior the night before.

"Don't you think you need to apologize, Dr. Leonard?" I asked.

"What for? I didn't *do* anything to you," he replied. "If there is a judgment to be made here, it is of you, not me."

"What for?" Jonathan asked in amazement.

"For not trying to stop me," he answered.

I was flabbergasted at this shift of focus from him to us, but my mind was on other matters as I strove to find the same satisfaction as Tony had found.

"I did try to stop you," Jonathan protested. "You shoved me aside and I knew I didn't stand a chance against you if I was to persist."

"Then I withdraw the judgment on you," Dr. Leonard said, "but it stands on everyone else."

"What about what you did to me?" I asked. "Don't you think I deserve an apology for *that*?"

"What did I do to you?"

I reminded him of our encounter in the kitchen, as well as the incident on the floor in his living room.

"I have no recollection of it, Ellen. Perhaps I was too drunk," he explained.

"Too drunk? You didn't look drunk at all," I answered.

He quickly explained how people can be inebriated without appearing so. Not everyone staggers or slurs their words when they're drunk, he said more with a tone of medical authority than in defense of his behavior. "I don't appear drunk when I am."

"Well, drunk or not," I insisted, "you owe me an apology." I needed something solid to come from this meeting.

"If I did what you say I did, then I do owe you an apology."

"I don't know about the kitchen incident," Jonathan offered, "but I can verify the living room incident."

"Then for that, I do apologize. What can I do to make it up to you?" He asked the question because it was the right thing to do, not because he was anxious to put right the things he had done. He had done much worse to me in the past, but those incidents had never evoked such a need for self-imposed justice. Those incidents, however, were without witnesses.

"I need time to think about it," I answered. This was all happening much too fast. And I was not prepared to deal with the lack of sincerity with which the question had been asked, nor with the aggravation at having to ask it.

"I'd really like to get this settled before Pat and I leave for our Christmas vacation. I want to put this behind me and feel free to enjoy myself while we're away." His frustration was apparent, as he intimated that I should have the answers when he wanted them.

"I'm sorry," I told him, "but I need some time."

"We'll take this up at your next session," he decided. He was certain that I would return.

I decided, during those intervening weeks, that in light of "the full context of everything" I knew about him, in light of his "overall character," and in light of the "benefit" he had been to me in therapy, I would accept his apology and would tell him so in the next session. I would also have to tell him, though, how shaken I was by that episode at his party and that we would have to discuss it before other matters could be discussed.

When that session arrived, he did not seem glad that I had accepted his apology without further explanation, nor did he seem relieved or grateful that I had chosen to ignore his offer for reparations. He seemed, rather, disinterested and bored. And when I discussed the effects that that night had on me and on my perception of him, he treated it the way he might have any other crisis in my life: shifting the focus from the event itself to my method of handling it, from his behavior to my disturbance over it. It was my childhood all over again.

We spoke of nothing else that hour, nothing else except how I felt as a patient watching him beat up another patient. It disturbed me when, at the end of the month, he billed me for that hour as if it had been no different from any other.

All the other party guests, Dr. Leonard said, received the same speech as Jonathan and I, save for the references to Dr. Leonard's behavior with me. And all of the party guests who were also his patients returned to their therapy with Dr. Leonard upon his return from vacation: each and every one of them.

10

THE ◇ BEACH
HOUSE

Therapy is generally considered to be a private and personal
process, with only the patient and the therapist being privy to
the contents of each session. Whereas Dr. Leonard insisted on
confidentiality from his patients, the same trust was often violated by the doctor himself.

On several occasions, Dr. Leonard would reveal to me "in
the strictest confidence" matters pertaining to other patient's
therapy, patients whom I knew. Once, for example, I was discussing a former acquaintance of mine with Dr. Leonard during
one of my sessions. Dr. Leonard took the opportunity to inform
me that this person had once been his patient. This disclosure
alone would have been considered a betrayal of a confidence by
most therapists, not to mention by the patient, but he went even
further than that.

It would have been "unethical," he told me, to explicitly
state the diagnosis he had made of his former patient, "but I can
do *this*." He proceeded to withdraw a textbook from the shelves,
the subject of which was sociopathic behavior patterns. Dr.
Leonard turned to its table of contents and instructed me to

skim it. Each chapter title was actually an identification of a symptom associated with the personality disorder. He pointed to several chapter titles, reading some of them aloud, and then asked, "Wouldn't you say this describes *Ira?*" It certainly did. Then he added that, since Ira had once been his patient, this insinuated diagnosis was to "be held in the strictest confidence."

On other occasions, I received similar, if not more explicit, diagnoses of his patients. "*Debbi's* problem is that she is incapable of accepting any kind of criticism." Or, the reason *Frank* was treating me strangely was "because one of Frank's problems is tremendous insecurity with women." Once, he even revealed the entire family background and situation of two of his patients. These incidents proved both reassuring and unsettling for me: reassuring because they told me that he trusted me; unsettling because he might feel equally inclined to discuss my therapy with others.

Just as Dr. Leonard held loosely the principles of confidentiality, so, too, did his patients violate the same restrictions placed on them. Such was the manner in which I first learned about *open sessions.*

Open sessions, my friends had told me, were therapy hours which had a predetermined beginning but no such ending. Once they had commenced, they were free to continue for as long as doctor and patient felt necessary. Because these sessions could last for as long as five or six hours, they were generally scheduled for Friday afternoons, the day on which Dr. Leonard scheduled no regular sessions and usually reserved for housecleaning, rest, or long weekends away.

The idea captured my attention and interest. It had been only a few weeks earlier when I dared to mention to Dr. Leonard my recent dissatisfaction over my progress in therapy.

"I feel like I have moved backwards," I told him. "I feel less in touch with myself than when I began therapy three years ago."

He looked at me with his bug eyes and shouted angrily, "What the hell have we been doing in here?"

He had taken my remark as a personal attack on his abilities, and I had not intended that. I quickly dropped the subject, claiming that "I am probably just feeling a little down today. Ignore what I said. I didn't mean it."

An open session, I reasoned, might produce some *real* progress, as well as indicate my continuing efforts to improve. I broached the subject with Dr. Leonard and his response was quite positive; we would have an open session.

He set the date for an upcoming Thursday night, not for a Friday afternoon as they usually were. Further, this session, he said, would take place not in his office, but at his girlfriend's beach house on the south Jersey shore. He had, he explained, already arranged for a long weekend there and didn't want to alter his plans. I accepted his terms, feeling grateful that he would see me at all.

I left for Point Pleasant, New Jersey, in the late afternoon. It was a long train ride, much longer than I had anticipated, and it was dark when I disembarked at the Point Pleasant station. Dr. Leonard was waiting for me in his Cadillac; he drove me the short distance to the beach house.

It was an incredibly tiny house. The kitchen, dining area, living area, and entry were all enclosed by a small rectangular room. There were two bedrooms, both of which opened directly off this multi-purpose room in which I was standing. Dr. Leonard took a seat at the table and invited me to sit across from him. There we remained for the next four hours.

It was an awkward time. I did not know exactly what to talk about, and he seemed disinterested in guiding me. I wanted to tell him again how I felt myself losing touch with my feelings and closing up. I wanted to say that, if intensity of feelings was a barometer of mental health, then I had gotten worse—much worse—since my therapy had begun. Sometimes I could feel nothing at all. But I said none of these things. I did not want to anger him.

I was disappointed at the conclusion of those four hours. My open session had included nothing more significant than superficial discussion revolving around current relationships in my life. Certainly, I thought, no progress was made here tonight.

Dr. Leonard rose to go to bed. He placed himself in between the entrances to the two bedrooms and pointed to the one on the left. "You can sleep there if you'd like," he offered. Then he added, "But I didn't put any sheets on the bed." He paused. "You *could* make it up if you *wanted* to."

Before I could reply that I had no objections to making up the bed myself, he continued. "Or, if you'd like to demonstrate your openness, you can sleep with me." Then he disappeared into the bedroom on the right.

I rose and walked to the midpoint between the two bedrooms. I stood there for a long time contemplating my choices. If I chose the unmade bed, I reasoned, he would interpret that as a sign of distrust and a lack of openness. I knew that would displease him, and I'd be certain to hear about it later. If I chose to sleep with him, he'd interpret that as a positive sign and be proud of me. Further, I considered, there was no longer any cause to fear sharing his bed. After all, he had vowed never to touch me again: not for the rest of his life. I chose to sleep in his bed.

I had been so long in making my decision that he had already turned out the lights and slipped into bed. Not certain if he had already fallen asleep, I quietly felt my way around until I found the edge of the bed. I lay down on top of the blanket and closed my eyes, hoping I had not awakened him.

"Aren't you going to undress?" he asked, disturbing the silence.

"No," I replied, "I don't think so."

"Ellen," he said, dragging out the sound of my name, "you're not pushing yourself."

"Okay," I answered. I did not want to debate this matter again. Besides, I thought, it is pitch black in here, and he isn't going to touch me anyway. I obeyed the implied command.

I lay down again, this time covering myself with the blanket.

I was on my back, remaining as close to the edge of this small bed as I could. I said "good-night" and closed my eyes to sleep.

"Would you mind rolling over?" he asked me. I thought he was asking for more room.

I rolled onto my right side, drawing my legs up toward my chest, and tried to inch even further toward the edge without falling off. Again, I said "good-night." He did not respond.

Within seconds, Dr. Leonard was grabbing me from behind, wrapping his arm firmly around my waist. He pushed himself up against my buttocks and, without difficulty or clumsiness, rammed his penis into my vagina. He moved only a few times and then ejaculated. The entire incident was over in less than half a minute.

He remained still for a moment, still keeping his penis inside of me. Then, without a word, he withdrew, and, putting his back to me, rolled over onto his left side to go to sleep.

I rolled over on my back and felt his semen draining from my body. Except for the burning sensation in my vagina, this was all I felt. I had gone numb. I had just been penetrated without consent, but I had no reaction. Not during the act nor after. This was what I had become: a woman who could feel no fear, no outrage, no indignation, no anger at being used. The fighter, the angry child I had once been was some other person I could barely remember. Now I had become someone who had lost her self and that left me in a vacuum of emotion. This was the product of my four years with Dr. Leonard: that I could feel nothing.

I stared at the ceiling calmly wondering what I would do if I got pregnant. I wasn't using birth control, and he, most assuredly, had not concerned himself with protection, either. The prospect didn't worry me. Nothing worried me. I just wondered about it. And with those thoughts, I fell asleep.

I waited until we were both wide awake and sipping the coffee he had made before I made any reference to last night's event.

"Why did you do that to me?" I asked him first. It was asked out of curiosity, not anger.

"Do what?" he answered.

"Why did you—penetrate me?"

He paused and then answered, "The trade is over, Ellen."

"What?"

"The trade is over," he repeated. "I won't answer that."

"What does that mean, *the trade is over?*" I asked.

"You think about it and come back to me when you think you understand," he replied.

Then he invited me out to breakfast, suggesting we leave an hour before my train was due. It was in the restaurant that I returned to the subject that was still on my mind.

"I thought you were never going to touch me again," I began.

"I always reserve the right to change my mind," he answered with a chuckle.

"Well, what does it mean that you did? I mean, what does it mean that, after all these years of not touching me, you had intercourse with me?" Once again, I was on a mission looking for answers.

"Ellen," he replied impatiently, "the trade is over. I am not going to answer these questions!"

"Remember when you told me that the only reason you weren't 'fucking' me was because I hadn't 'earned that sanction yet'?"

He nodded in recognition of his words.

"What did I do to earn that sanction now?" I asked.

"The—trade—is—over," he repeated. He spoke his words slowly and adamantly.

"But I want to know why you did that to me last night!" My voice had grown louder as I struggled for some understanding. I was not angry. I was, again, confused.

"Quiet!" he ordered. "This is not the place to be discussing what happened last night. Let's drop it."

I was quiet for a moment while I considered his words, *the trade is over.* Could he, I wondered, mean *trade* in the merchant sense of the word? Does he see last night as some kind of exchange of goods!? Does he believe we had some sort of con-

121

tract which specified that I would give him something in return for something he would give me?

I knew enough not to pose my hypothesis to him now. More questioning on this matter would only anger him further. When I presented my interpretation to him at my next session, however, he confirmed it, adding, ". . . and once the goods have been exchanged, you can't go back and ask for a clarification of the terms."

"When was this contract made?" I asked him next. "And what were the goods that I received?"

"The trade is over, Ellen. Let's move on," he would only say. He would answer me in this way every time I questioned him on that night's activity.

I finished my breakfast in silence and waited for him to suggest we leave. When he reached for the check, I asked him one last question.

"Does this mean I am off probation?"

"Yes, Ellen," he chuckled, "you're off probation."

I pushed out of my mind the issues I felt stirring within me, as I rode the train back to Manhattan. I read part of a book I had carried with me, and even managed to catch a nap. By the time I reached the city, my questions had been sufficiently suppressed and I was feeling better. I had not yet realized what a profound and long-term impact that night would have on me, but I was to experience the beginning of its effects before that day was over.

Upon my arrival home, I immediately telephoned Jonathan, whom I had stopped dating some months earlier, and asked to see him that evening after he had finished work. I knew what I was calling him for, but I made no connection in my mind between my motives now and the events of last night.

When he arrived at my apartment shortly after six, I wasted no time in inviting him to my bedroom. There, I seduced him and, for his pleasure alone, we had sexual intercourse. When it was over, I politely asked him to leave, explaining that I had other plans for the rest of the night.

He had not been gone more than ten minutes when I reached for the telephone again, this time to request the company of a married man from my office to whom I had been quite attracted. He was still at the office when I called, and eagerly agreed to visit me that night. It did not concern me that I had already had sex with two other men in less than twenty-four hours, or that he was married, or that I felt no desire now. I was simply determined to sleep with him that night. And I did.

Eric was spending the night at a friend's home, so my time was my own to do as I pleased. Doing so marked the beginning of a two-month affair with a married man, and the beginning of almost a two-year period of promiscuity. I slept with single men and married men, older men and younger men. I accepted almost any proposition that came my way, as I felt no right in saying "no," and I propositioned the rest. As long as I found him minimally attractive, any man was a candidate for the bedroom. Even those I found repulsive, I thought about twice before turning them down.

It was not pleasure I was seeking, as oftentimes I was sickened by the encounter and vomited afterward. At the best of times, I excused myself and went to the bathroom, where I would sob. Yet I compulsively sought out new partners, while at the same time, dissuading any man who had more *honorable* intentions. It was this switching back and forth between indiscriminate pursuit and the sickness that followed that provided the first glimmer of another change that was brewing inside me. I seemed to be developing two personalities.

This was not a case of multiple personalities, as it is classically known; I was totally aware of both parts of me, as well as which mode I was operating in at any given time. That, however, was *all* I understood about them at the time. I was aware that some sort of schism was occurring within me, but it seemed to be without cause or reason. The fact that it suddenly began upon my return from the Jersey shore went completely unnoticed.

123

I referred to one part of myself as *me* and to the other part as *her*, or *Big Me* and *Little Me*, respectively, as Dr. Leonard came to call them. They were called such because of their tremendous age difference. *I*, or *Big Me*, was twenty-five years old and functioned solely in an adult world. *She*, or *Little Me*, functioned in a regressed stage of childhood, rarely exceeding the age of seven. Their beginnings, however, were so subtle that their first appearances seemed unnoteworthy.

Big Me had begun her emergence before I had even returned to Manhattan. While riding the train from Point Pleasant, I had experienced no anxiety, guilt, or depression. While lying in his bed that night, there had been no anger, tears, or turmoil. That was the first time that sex with my therapist had produced such an absence of negative reactions. With this change, *I*, or Big Me, was born. The night of my return home, after my married man had left the apartment, I felt myself withdrawing into myself, unable to speak, and only able to cry. Finding comfort in the company of a doll, I curled up with it under the covers of my bed, and hid from the world. With this, *she*, or Little Me, was born.

At the time, *I* felt that a real sign of progress had been made. Having rid myself of all the negative emotions that had surrounded my encounters with Dr. Leonard, I had clearly moved in the direction he had prescribed for me. *She*, however, was seen as nothing more significant than a passing depression. I was wrong on both counts.

As days passed, and then weeks, *she* made *her* presence known with more frequency and greater intensity, and *she* lasted for longer periods of time, as well. *She* began to experience herself as separate from the other part of me, as *she* withdrew deeper and deeper. Concurrently, *I* experienced *her* presence as an annoyance, as *she* was what blocked my way to a clean bill of health. Each, therefore, was comfortable labeling the other a separate entity.

I was the intellectual half, doing all of our thinking and reasoning. *She* was the emotional counterpart, doing all of *our* feeling and emoting. Each, unknown to me at the time, was representing her function in the purest form, with Big Me capable of no real feelings, and Little Me capable of no conceptual thought.

I was the one who came to represent the roles of femininity and sexuality as Dr. Leonard had taught them—in his bedroom and in his office. *I* spouted his ideas, *I* integrated their meanings into my behavior, and *I* took them to their logical conclusions. Engaging in multiple sexual relationships, telling my therapist that *I* loved and desired him, and ceasing my remaining challenges to his lectures and sexual treatment of me, *I* became the paragon of *Sexual Psychology according to Leonard*. As such, he invited me to dine with him, at his expense, in exchange for the opportunity to "pick (my) brain": he was gathering supportive data on his *Polygamous Nature of Women* theory. He not only approved of me, he now considered me a worthy source of information on feminine psychology.

And just as *I* had embodied the knowledge given to me in discussion with my therapist, so did *I* embody the lesson he had taught me in bed: to seek fulfillment by and pleasure in being used.

In the second year of Big Me and Little Me, *I* slowly developed a new symptom unique to only Big Me. After several weeks of dieting to drop ten pounds, I began to restrict my caloric intake to under three hundred calories a day—and I began to induce vomiting. I did not disclose this ritual to Dr. Leonard, nor to anyone else for that matter. It was not that I was hiding what I considered to be a serious problem. It was that I did not consider this eating disorder to be a problem at all. After all, I was getting better, I was in control, I was out of pain. I was becoming perfectly healthy.

She, or Little Me, on the other hand, was something else altogether. She came to represent all of that inside me that was truly me. *She* was the core of my being, the reality of my soul. Conceived in fear, *she* embodied all the feelings that had been shunned, discouraged, and punished by my therapist whenever they had been expressed in my adult form. The form she took, therefore, was that of a child.

Unable to articulate *her* doubts, *her* confusions, and *her* needs, *she* posed no threat to Dr. Leonard; therefore, *she* was safe from his judgments. *Her* single function was to feel. *Her* single avenue of expression was through emoting. *She* was the regressed form of who I had come to bury with Dr. Leonard.

Almost perpetually in pain, *she* did little else than sit in silence or cry. *She* withdrew inside herself where she usually remained for hours, sometimes for days. When *she* was the predominating personality, *we* would go for that long without ever speaking a word.

And when it was time for a session, it was *she* who would usually emerge. She sought the comfort and security of the paternal embrace of her therapist who had come to recognize *her* appearance. There, for the moment of her session's hour, she would be cradled and rocked as Dr. Leonard tried to soothe this little girl who ached so.

On some of those occasions when it was *she* who arrived for a therapy session and not *I*, she might burst into tears immediately upon entering his office. Not able to identify or articulate *her* pain, *she* would just wait for Dr. Leonard to beckon *her* to the floor where he would hug *her* and whisper that everything would be all right. Often, on Dr. Leonard's instruction, *she* carried her doll with *her* to the session when being without it was too difficult. Dr. Leonard encouraged this "prop," as he felt that anything that kept *her* with him aided him in the psychotherapeutic process to unravel the mystery of *her* source.

He urged *her* to continue crying, whispering, "Let it out, let it all out." He rocked *her* and stroked *her* for nearly the whole hour *she* spent with him. He knew *she* could not speak, so he rarely asked *her* questions for fear of losing *her* to *me*. Then, sometimes, before the session would end, he would remove her clothes. On one occasion, while the videotape was recording, while *she* lay crying on the floor clinging to her doll, while he still whispered words of comfort, he rolled on top of *her* and penetrated *her*.

126

Once, he undressed *her* for something other than intercourse. Having removed his clothes first and then *hers* at the beginning of the hour, he concluded the session by pressing his penis against *her* belly and moving until he ejaculated. He cleaned both of them off, turned off the recorder, and sent *her* home.

Following these sessions, *she* would retreat further behind the doll and the silence. Sometimes it would take a full day or more before *I* could reemerge to touch base with reality. Most times, however, *I* arrived several hours after such a session had ended. Either way, whenever *I* appeared, my behavior was most predictable. Each time, *I* found myself pursuing a new bed partner for that night.

Whereas I took great care during this time to not expose my son to the parade of sex partners through his mother's life, I had much less control over his witness to Little Me. On those occasions when it was Little Me whom he found waiting for him at the end of a school day, when not enough time had elapsed between my session and his return home, it was all I could do to just place his afternoon snack on the table. Then I would point to my throat and explain away my inability to speak with faked illness. After the emergence of Little Me took on a pattern consistent with the timing of my therapy sessions, though, I began to make after-school arrangements for Eric *just in case.* Once every other week, he would play with his classmates at their home, and on the off-week we would return the invitation. On the occasions during those two years when Little Me remained predominant for longer than a day, I reverted to the sickness excuse to explain my silence, and pushed myself to tend to his needs. Making his supper, giving him his bath, required all the effort and energy I had within me. But at the end of the day, at the arrival of my son's bedtime, I knew that, once again, I could take refuge in the solitude of my bed and the comfort of my doll. I don't believe Eric ever sensed anything more wrong than that his Mommy was feeling ill.

During these two years that I vacillated between Big Me and Little Me, I struggled to find some clue that might explain this phenomenon. Dr. Leonard hypothesized that *she* was the part of me that found it easier to retreat than to be healthy. *She*, he posited, was afraid of therapy ever coming to an end.

I did not understand until many years later how wrong he was. It was *I* who had surrendered, while *she* had remained the keeper of my spirit.

Sometime after my visit to Point Pleasant, I stopped working. I had had a good job with a department-store chain, but had found myself increasingly unable to handle the management position after the beach house incident, though there had been no problem before. I became restless. I experienced guilt over working while Eric was greeted by babysitters after school. I couldn't concentrate, and told myself that it was due to neglected parental responsibilities at home. Whatever the true cause, I quit and felt relief at the diminished pressure in my life.

Much of the therapy for Big Me was still concerned with questions from my past and unresolved feelings with which it had left me. Had I really been singled out by my mother, or had I *misperceived* the events of my youth? Had there really been hatred in my mother's eyes, or had I *misinterpreted* her message? Had I reason to be so confused by her behavior, or was my confusion the product of a deeper disturbance within me? The answers came from my mother herself during a phone conversation in the spring of 1976.

I had telephoned Mommy in Chicago to ascertain flight information for a trip we were all to make to New Orleans in May. It was to be a celebration of my father's fiftieth birthday, and he wanted to take his whole family on a three-day holiday for the occasion. (I guess when my father made travel plans for *his* "whole family," he meant to include me.) I told Mommy of the purpose of my call, explaining that my ex-husband was to watch Eric while I was in New Orleans, and that David needed the exact departure and return dates. But I never received the information for which I had phoned.

"Just think, if you were still married to David, you wouldn't have this problem," she said sarcastically.

"Mom, could you just give me the flight information?" I retorted. But I could already sense that the conversation was headed for trouble. I sensed it as soon as she heard my voice.

Within minutes, the conversation had taken an irreversible turn.

"You're disgusting," she said to me. She said it with an icy coldness that made it sound like fact, not opinion. "You turn my stomach, Ellen—and you always have!" she proclaimed. She was being liberated from something in this conversation, and there was no stopping her now.

"Why are you doing this, Mom?" I asked her, holding back my tears.

"I can't remember a time when I could stand the sight of you. You've always made me sick!" she continued without losing control or coldness. "I hate you. I hate everything you are, everything you've always been—and I can't remember a time when I didn't."

She was delivering the same fury and hostility I had witnessed so many times before, but this time it was not in shrieks and screams, it was in words and intensity. She meant what she was saying, and we both knew it.

"I have to hang up now, Mother. I can't listen to you anymore," I told her, still trying to contain my tears.

Addressing my emerging tears more than my words, she answered, "What's the matter, Ellen? Are you going to tell me that you didn't know this before?"

I could not answer her. Of course I had felt it before, I had sensed it before, I had thought it before. But I guess I never really *knew* it before. I had never been ready to know it before. I wasn't ready now, either, but this time I could not escape it.

"I'm hanging up now, Mother," I forewarned her. I could not just hang up on my mother.

"What's wrong? Can't take it?" she asked, still trying to engage me in more of this attack.

"Good-bye, Mother," I said on the verge of tears before I hung up.

I knew I would not be going to New Orleans. And I knew we had just spoken for the last time.

When I broke down and sobbed at the conversation's end, it was not Little Me who was crying, but every part of who I was: the little girl of my childhood, the twenty-five-year-old woman of my adulthood, and the adolescent who bridged the two. I cried as much for the pain her words had caused me, as I did for all the unnecessary confusion that had consumed so much of my childhood. I cried less for the loss of a mother, than for the loss of hope that she would ever be the mother I wanted. And I cried in relief and recognition of the fact that the perceptions of my childhood had not been evidence of any insanity, but of my sensitivity to and awareness of the reality around me.

It was several weeks later when I received the phone call from my father that closed the door on our relationship, as well.

"I'm calling to find out why you haven't called your mother in the last few weeks. Is it because of that little spat she told me she had with you on the phone?" he asked. His mood was angry, his tone abrupt.

"Daddy, I have a date here right now. Could I call you back on this later?" I had quickly sensed from the harshness in his voice that this would be a conversation that should not be conducted with company sitting just feet away.

"Just a *yes* or *no* will do. You don't have to call me back."

"Daddy, I don't know what she told you, but that was no 'little spat' we had over . . ."

"Just *yes* or *no*. Have you not called her because of that little spat?" he demanded again. "Do you know that your mother just had surgery? She is very hurt that you didn't call her to find out how she was feeling. Do you know that?"

She was hurt! After what she said to me on the phone, she was hurt? I didn't know whether to laugh or scream, but I was beginning to see why Daddy had really called. He was not interested in a dialogue or in receiving answers to his questions. He

was barely giving me room to respond. He had
me and to pass sentence. Now I knew what the
be and I started to fight for my father.

"I know she was supposed to have surg
wasn't dangerous surgery and . . ."

"So you deliberately did not call her. Is that rig..
asked, already knowing the answer.

"Daddy, would you like to hear what she said to me during
our so-called *little spat?*" I asked hoping that he would, but
certain that he would not.

"You've answered my question, Ellen." Then he pronounced judgment. "You have no sense of loyalty! None. Not
even for your own mother."

We had heard much about *loyalty* growing up. It was one of
three topics on family living with which Daddy was well versed.
No matter what, no matter what was done to us, above all else,
our loyalty to our mother was expected. And when we fell short
of those expectations, it was demanded. I did not understand
that duty then. I understood it even less now.

The second topic on which he was an expert was on parents
not apologizing to their children. Often I heard Daddy say that,
even if Mommy *punished* us and should not have, "she doesn't
have to apologize. She's your mother." The same exemption
applied to him, as well. The rule was made clear from as far
back as I can remember: parents *never* apologize to their children.

But the last topic was my father's specialty, for no one but
him was in a position to issue such a lecture and have me even
consider the possibility of its veracity. Whenever my mother's
hostility, my father's obedience to her, and my confusion had
seemed to be overwhelming my life, my father would witness
my rage and dictate his warning.

"Ellen," he would say impatiently and sternly, "this family is
no worse than any other." He meant it. "In fact, it's better than
most. You could have done a hell of a lot worse. And if you
don't see that, it's only because other families hide what's really

ng on. They present a rosy picture to the outside world. But
at picture isn't reality. On the inside, they're all suffering."

My mother had frequently issued the same lecture, but the
source allowed me to ignore the content. When my father spoke
these words, however, they came from the adult to whom I
looked for rationality, sanity, and answers. So I considered his
words. Contemplated their possibility. And then dismissed
them. It was not that I distrusted Daddy that kept me from believing these words. I simply could not accept that the whole
world existed the way we did inside our apartment walls. Such
suffering was not only too awesome for a little girl to consider, it
also meant I would never find a way out.

"The only thing left to say is that if you won't talk to your
mother, then you're no daughter of mine." He did not say
good-bye. He just slammed the receiver into the cradle of the
phone and our conversation was terminated. So was our relationship.

As tumultuous and traumatic as my life frequently felt with Big
Me, Little Me, and the termination of the relationship with my
parents, so it was equally nourished and sustained by the increasingly pleasurable relationship with my son, and the deepening and developing relationship with two friends, Tony and
Linda, respectively.

Tony and I had shared company regularly, if not frequently,
since the Christmas party at Dr. Leonard's home two years earlier, and though he was not privy to the secrets of Little Me, or
the history of my relationship with our therapist, or my daily
rituals of induced vomiting, I did feel free to share almost all
the other intimacies of my life with him. He, it seemed, felt the
same, as we sat over endless pots of coffee exchanging the news
of our lives, the stories of our pasts, and the hopes for our fu-
tures. A total lack of chemistry, however, precluded the expan-
sion of our friendship into a romance, and that was always
understood by us both. Whatever communication and affection
there was between us passed in deep friendship.

Linda had been introduced to me through mutual friends years earlier, but it was not until 1976 that our relationship blossomed into the closest friendship that I had ever shared with a woman. She, too, was a patient of Dr. Leonard, and echoed my words of admiration and respect for our therapist. We spent endless hours in conversation, and just as many hours in backgammon games, theaters, and New York restaurants. We shared many more interests than Tony and I shared, so often our friendship found us like two sisters exploring the world around them. We rejoiced in the love and sense of discovery which we were each experiencing for the first time in a relationship with a woman, and our excitement with what we had found in one another was evident to all who knew us.

As close and open as my friendship was with Linda, I did not disclose to her either the existence of Little Me or the cause of my continued weight loss. But she did see a side of me that Tony did not—the side that a woman can only show to another woman: how it feels to be in bed with a man you love; how it feels to be in bed with a man you don't; how it feels to be lonely for a man you can love when all the men you seem to know aren't worth knowing; who you couldn't sleep with even if he were the last man on earth; who you wouldn't sleep with now, but might sleep with if he were the last man on earth. And whenever a disclosure was finished, we each felt totally understood because we knew that the other was just like her.

My friends were my sustenance, my place of refueling. Especially Linda. I felt wanted, understood, and loved by her. Those feelings were reciprocated. And when all else might be going awry in my day, I always knew I could lean on Linda for support. But it was both of my friends who came to be a family for me, and I counted on both of them the way I had always wished I could count on my own.

As my relationships were deepening elsewhere, my relationship with my therapist hit a snag. Starting in the spring of 1976, he began experiencing difficulty in getting *her* to appear before him. Up till then, *she* had appeared regularly and without prompting. Whereas *she* continued to emerge with regularity *after* my sessions were over, resistance to Dr. Leonard's presence grew stronger.

It was around the time of my conversation with my mother that Dr. Leonard first noticed the trouble he had in getting *her* to appear before him, but it was not until early December of 1976 that he conducted the first of two consecutive sessions in my apartment "in order to make *her* more comfortable with the surroundings." An environment equipped with familiar "props," such as the blanket *she* hid under or the nightgown that was the only outfit clearly distinguished as *her* own, might facilitate *her* emergence, he reasoned.

He instructed me to wear the nightgown, hide under the blanket, and hold the doll, for at least an hour before this home-session. Perhaps, he hoped, *she* would be ready to visit with him when he arrived. I made after-school arrangements for Eric and followed my doctor's instructions.

Upon entering my apartment, Dr. Leonard announced that the session would be conducted in the bedroom—*her* hiding place. There, he immediately disrobed and climbed on the bed. He extended his arm, indicating that I should let him hold me, the way he held *her*.

I cuddled in his arms and tried to feel the emergence of Little Me, but *she* was not cooperating.

"Suck on my nipples," he ordered, "then tell me if it makes you feel anything that reminds you of when you were a baby."

"I wasn't breast-fed, Dr. Leonard."

"Try it anyway," he urged.

With embarrassment and uneasiness, I followed his orders.

"Tell me what you're feeling," he said.

"Nothing," I replied, interrupting the activity he had commanded. "Absolutely nothing. This is dumb."

"Then come lie on top of me and let me rock you," he was now suggesting more gently.

"Just rock me like this," I responded, only wanting to be lightly held and comforted.

"You can't get close enough that way," he argued, and playfully—as if I were his little girl—pulled me on top of his naked body.

There he kept me until the session was over. When some time had passed and all he continued to do was rock me back and forth, I began to relax. I closed my eyes after a while and felt the warmth of his hug, the soothing motion of the rocking, and the sense of protection that only a little girl can feel. It was not Little Me I was feeling, as there was no pain, no withdrawal. It was just the little girl part of me that had lingered into adulthood.

When my hour was over, he looked at his watch and told me it was time for him to dress. I was sorry he was leaving just then, as I had almost been lulled to sleep by the rolling motion and the soft words he had continued to speak during this hug. He rolled me off him, onto my back. He left the bed, but he did not proceed to dress.

Standing over me now, he lifted my nightgown and removed my underwear. Then, placing one knee on the bed, he put his penis up to my vagina and asked, "Are you using birth control?" He had never asked me before; I did not know why he was bothering now.

"No," I answered, somewhat startled. "I use foam."

With that, he quickly pulled back, never having penetrated me, and ran to the bathroom. When he returned, he carried with him my cannister of spermicide and the applicator. He filled it and inserted the dosage into my vagina. He repeated this procedure a second time, and then prepared for his departure in silence.

It was only three days later when he returned for another try at getting to *her*. Again, he disrobed, asking, "How close is *she* today?"

He did not ask me to suck on his nipples, nor did he want me to lie on his body. He did less talking this hour than he had during the last, as "it might have been all those instructions that scared her off."

I waited like that for an hour, trying very hard to feel *her* presence in the quiet of the room; but *she* remained hidden. Dr. Leonard checked his watch, and then stood to dress without speaking a word. After he had put on only his shirt, he returned to the edge of the bed where, once again, he stood over me. And, as he had done a few days before, he placed one knee on the bed, pulled my hips toward him, removed my underclothes, and penetrated me for just the few seconds it took him to ejaculate. Then, without any word about birth control, without any word at all, he finished dressing and left.

Neither Dr. Leonard nor I knew it yet, but that was to be the last time he would ever touch me.

11

THE CONFRONTATION

December 1976–May 1977

It had been exactly five years since the beginning of my therapy, one year and eight months since my visit to the beach house, and three weeks since my last home session, when a complication in my personal life caused renewed anxiety and apprehension in my therapy. I had just turned twenty-six when I began to fall in love. Unexpected, unplanned, and unwanted, this new development necessarily resulted in a turmoil that felt all too familiar to me.

I was formally introduced to Tony's brother, Greg, toward the end of December. It was a meeting markedly different from all the others I had had during the previous two years, but then this man seemed different from all the others I had met during that time. There was a gentleness in his eyes, the likes and degree of which I had never seen before. And they sparkled, too. He was soft-spoken, laid back, and unassuming in his presence. Yet there was a strength in his face that kept my eyes riveted on him as I tried to figure out if it was coming from self-confidence, or from past experiences and old wounds, or both. His tall stance and lean muscular build only added to the excitement I felt in his presence. I found myself yearning to be near him and subtly vying for his attention.

We talked until the last hours of darkness, that first night we met. I knew well before dawn that I had discovered something special, and I was as excited by that knowledge as I was by the man himself.

There was rarely a night or weekend that we did not spend together after that initial introduction. My feelings for Greg grew quickly and strong. And whether it was his lack of typical male aggressiveness, which I had come to expect and reluctantly tolerate, or the undivided attention I received from him, or the specialness with which he treated me, I knew that monogamy and romance went hand-in-hand for this man who was also a patient of Dr. Leonard. To question me on that assumption would never have entered his mind.

"Promise me," I begged Greg often, "promise me that you'll always stay just like you are and never try to become like Dr. Leonard."

"What do you mean?" he would answer.

It always surprised me that he didn't understand what I meant. How, I wondered, did he ever escape the influence and information of Dr. Leonard's theories on masculinity and feminity? "Just promise that no matter how long you stay with Dr. Leonard, you'll never become like him. His patients always become like him, but I don't want you any different than the way you are."

"I promise," he answered in bewilderment. "I have no intention of ever being anyone other than who I am."

I knew an end had come to the one-night stands and brief affairs. I would not want to risk losing what I had just found. I knew, too, that an end must come to the episodes of five-second intercourse with my therapist, and that I would have to tell Dr. Leonard that.

I had planned a speech nearly five years ago similar to the one I was planning now. This time, however, it was harder. This time, I would not be able to explain to him why I felt my choice for monogamy to be the right one. Intellectually, I would be unable to dispute his theories, for my actions now were based only on feelings, not reason. Emotionally, I felt guilt over acting on premises from an old "unhealthy psychology," rather than forcing myself to act on the new and healthy ideas that he had taught me. But it was a speech I was determined to give, nevertheless.

I rehearsed my words for the week preceding my first session of 1977. I tried different phrases, different tones of voice, different approaches. I sought the combination that would serve to minimize the anger and the impatience I expected to see when I made my announcement to him. I wrote down several speeches, and tried to memorize the one I thought was best. I spoke the words into a tape recorder, looking for ways of improving—making softer—the message I had to deliver. None of these lessened my fear; I hoped only that they would lessen his fury.

"Greg is very special to me," I started out nervously on this January 4th session. "He's just not like any of the others, and I don't want to push him away."

Dr. Leonard had expressed concern during previous sessions about my compulsion to sleep with so many different men. He wondered what was causing it and analyzed on occasion that it might stem from a fear of getting close to any one man. "If you sleep with men that don't matter to you, you, in effect, *push away* the ones who might," he had said. That was my intention, I had replied.

I took a deep breath and came right to the point. Softly I said, "I don't think I want to sleep with anyone else except him."

There was silence in the office. I drew my stare from my lap and met his eyes which were fixed on my face. He was waiting for me to say something further, as if he didn't know that I had finished. I waited a few seconds more for him to ask me a question. Then I broke the silence.

". . . and that includes you, Dr. Leonard."

He quickly grew impatient and exasperated. "What's brought this on, may I ask?"

I was scared. I did not want to answer by telling him that Greg made me feel important and feminine, for that would imply that Dr. Leonard did not. I did not want to confess that Greg was the only man with whom I experienced real pleasure, for that would confirm an absence of it with Dr. Leonard, a most unhealthy symptom, at best. I could not tell him how much I enjoyed and needed the tenderness I received from Greg—in and out of the bedroom—for the absence of it from my therapist told me that those needs were unnecessary and illegitimate for healthy people. I did not want to tell him that sex with Greg had never involved instructions, orders, or intimidation, for that was not the standard I had learned from Dr. Leonard. And I could not tell him how I relished the long talks with Greg after we had made love, for Dr. Leonard had always found my need for discourse an annoyance. It was not my therapist whom I tried to spare from these comparisons. It was his two patients, Greg and me. I could not bring myself to explain that one of his male patients behaved so contrary to the behavior of our perfectly healthy therapist, and that I, his paragon of sexual adjustment, enjoyed it.

"I don't think Greg would understand," was all I could think to say. "And it's not worth the risk of losing him."

The tension left his face, and the anger disappeared from his eyes. Then he smiled slightly. "We'll see," was his only remark.

In the first two months of therapy that followed, my sessions reverted to the superficial level of current event discussions that had once before filled the days of off-limit subjects and unresolved dilemmas. For reasons that I could not comprehend at the time, Dr. Leonard stopped conducting derepression sessions. He no longer prompted me to lie on the floor in order to search for hidden emotions, or insist that I appear naked in front of him in order to effect more productive therapy hours. Instead, he asked me questions about my present life, the college courses for which I was currently registered, career plans for the future, and occasionally, the status of my relationship with Greg. And for each of those sessions, he remained in the doctor's chair fully clothed, while I sat across the desk from him in the patient's chair the same way.

The closest he came to disrupting the facade of peace that had come to rest between us was when he questioned me during one February session on the inherent contradiction between the ideas I had previously accepted from him and the happiness I now appeared to have found in a romance that conflicted with those views. When he asked how I reconciled the two, I answered, and he wrote down, that I operated on two different levels: "(1) what I know in my head and (2) what I feel." My behavior with Greg was the result of the latter. He pursued the matter no further.

The days of Big Me and Little Me seemed to have waned during this time without my ever really knowing when or why. It was sometime in March when I was first aware of *her* long absence from my life. Not only had *she* long since given up appearing in front of Dr. Leonard, *she* now ceased emerging in the privacy of my own apartment, as well. And in the tranquility, security, and happiness of my new romance, I stopped trying to figure out why *she* had ever come in the first place, and seemed not to care any longer about the reason she had initially developed. All that mattered now was my time with Greg.

In March and April, my sessions grew rockier. For the first time in over five years, I found myself disagreeing and arguing with my therapist. The issue of our battle: sex.

"How the hell is a woman expected to enjoy sex if she never gets touched?" I barged in demanding one afternoon. I had not even waited for him to be seated before my anger came rushing out. I was not referring so much to how he had interacted with me in the bedroom, as I was to his lectures which explicitly taught me to strive for orgasms without any tactile stimulation.

He had often repeated that such "foreplay should not be neces-sary" for the healthy woman.

Without batting an eye, he took a seat, turned on the video recorder, and calmly asked, "What's this?"

"I thought there was something wrong with me for wanting to be touched during sexual play. *You* taught me that! You taught me that *all* my pleasure should come from what I do to my partner, that a healthy woman should not need direct stim-ulation, touching, kissing—*anything!* Well, that's not true," I said with certainty and anger. "It's just not true."

As I spoke, I could easily have been referring to Dr. Leonard's sexual style in bed, but I was not and he knew it. That would have been a riskier criticism, a more personal judg-ment than what I was prepared to make. We both knew there had never been any preliminary sex play: not before his request-ing fellatio, not before his penetrating me. There had never been so much as a kiss. Except for his penis, he had never used any part of his body to touch me in a sexual manner, save for the first night in his bed when he painfully kneaded my breasts while calling for me to fight. Had objection to his sexual style been my present focus, we both knew I would never have said so; he, because such topics had been placed off-limits long ago, and I, because fear of his anger precluded personal judgments that were certain to provoke it.

I had been set free, for this first of many outbursts, by a chain of events. The pleasure in my relationship with Greg, his encouragement to be free with myself and his eagerness to have our lovemaking a mutually enjoyable venture, reminded me by contrast of the nagging questions about the past with Dr. Leonard that had never been answered. The security I found in my relationship with Greg freed me to pursue this apparent con-flict. I headed to the bookstore for data and then to my best girl-friend, Linda, for corroboration.

Linda, too, was Dr. Leonard's patient, and she faced the same resistance to challenging his ideas as I. But two going at it was easier than one alone, and the printed information helped pave the way. By the time I had finished the research on my own and the dialogues with my friend, the answers were coming in loud and clear: I was not alone in what I was needing. I was not neurotic in what I was wanting. I was perfectly normal. And the revelation stunned and angered me.

My therapist listened to me intently. He did not look angry, impatient, or exasperated. Instead, he took the pose of a student under instruction from a teacher.

"I am only a healthy male," he explained half apologetically. "I can only introspect about what is necessary for a healthy male. Women, on the other hand, I must learn about through women—healthy women. If they don't tell me, how am I supposed to know?"

"You're a doctor. I expect you to know! And if you don't know, you shouldn't be pretending that you do!"

"What have you been learning?" he asked.

I gave him the titles of the books I had bought and suggested that he read them himself, on his own time rather than on my therapy time.

"What if I paid you for a session? Would you be willing to teach me what you've learned?" He was dead serious. He wanted to know what I knew.

Still angry at the misinformation I had been fed, I declined.

Subsequent sessions were similar. Each time I finished reading a new article or book, each time I finished another conversation with Linda on this topic, my anger was refueled, and I marched into my next session with even more furor than the last time.

"How the hell could you teach Female Sexuality for the last five years and never once, in all that time, mention the word *clitoris*?"

"What would you have liked me to say about it?" was his quiet, gentle reply. He was baiting me into *teaching* him again. He was disarming me, as well, and my anger was quickly dissipating. I thought, He really does want to know. I believed his naïveté and ignorance. So I told him about what I had read, and about what Linda and I verified through one another. And I told him that it all confirmed what I had always felt to be true about my own body, but which he had been teaching me to change and view as unhealthy.

I cannot say for how long these sessions might have continued had they not been interrupted by an unforeseen and unrelated event. I was experiencing anger over what Dr. Leonard had *taught* me—in the office and in the bedroom—not over what he had *done* to me, when a telephone call from Tony one cool night early in May brought about an abrupt change in my focus.

There was a sense of urgency in Tony's voice, as he requested to see me within the hour. The crisis I sensed brewing was further confirmed by Tony's request that I ask Greg to leave the apartment we were now sharing so that we could have a conversation in private. This was not typical of Tony, as he had never, in over two years of friendship, phoned me in such a manner. We had certainly, on occasion, shared some of our problems, but rarely did the topics extend beyond the trouble he was experiencing with a girlfriend or the problems I had had with my parents. We had never sought each other out during a personal crisis: Tony seemed to have none, and mine could not be discussed. This time, however, would be different.

He did not speak a word, nor did he so much as glance in my direction, as he passed by where I was standing to greet him at the door. His face was tense, drawn, and pained, as he quickly found his way to a chair at my dining room table and waited for me to join him. He remained silent until I was seated across from him, and then he began.

He stumbled over his opening words, looking for the right way to tell me what he had come to say. He stared at the table top, starting his first sentence again and again, until he knew that no easy way would deliver this message, so the painful way would have to do. "Someone told me," he finally stated, "that Dr. Leonard had sexual intercourse with her during one of her sessions."

144

My body stiffened, my face tightened, and my gaze, too, now dropped to the dining room table. I knew I could not enter into this discussion without the threat of being expelled from therapy, and I was immediately panic-stricken. I could not think. I could not speak. My mind was racing, but no thought seemed to endure long enough for contemplation.

Tony did not seem to notice my reaction, as he was still too preoccupied with what he had heard that day. Still fixated on the table top, he continued to speak, filling me in on all of the details he had been given by one of Dr. Leonard's former patients.

He told me how Dr. Leonard had asked her for back rubs and how that had eventually led to his having her masturbate and fellate him. He told me that Dr. Leonard had forced her to undress for derepression sessions at the threat of not continuing them at all, and how he had video-recorded her lying naked in a spread-eagle position. He told me how Dr. Leonard, at the end of one of her sessions, had watched her crawl into a fetal position to help hide the nakedness that was so discomforting, and how he had used that opportunity to take her from behind by surprise, penetrating her vagina.

I was both sickened by this account of what could have been my own experience, and paralyzed by my fear at being party to its revelation. I wondered why hearing his treatment of another woman was so repulsive, when that same treatment of me had only evoked self-doubts, guilt, and anxiety. I wondered why his treatment of her was so nauseating, but his treatment of me had become my standard for mental health. I wondered why I felt that she was victimized, but that I was *sanctioned* by the same behavior. My body began to tremble, as I struggled in vain to control the eruption rumbling inside me.

Tony was still not looking at me when he asked, "Do you think it could be true? I don't see how it could be. But why would she say those things? Maybe she's just out to get Dr. Leonard for some sick reason." He thought about that for a minute and then added, "But she didn't appear to be doing that when I spoke to her." Then he looked up for my response.

He caught my eyes moving away from his, as I searched for something I could say without getting into trouble. "Maybe she just wasn't healthy enough to understand what he was doing to her, Tony," was all that came to mind to say.

"What?" Tony asked incredulously.

"If Dr. Leonard did do this, Tony, maybe someday she'll be feminine enough to understand it." I was trying to defend what I knew to be true about Dr. Leonard without acknowledging the validity of the story. I was trying to put an end to this discussion without ever really getting involved in it. And I was trying not to show that I was scared to death.

There was a long moment of silence. Then Tony's face slowly moved from tension to pained compassion as he gently and lovingly asked, "How long has Dr. Leonard been doing this to *you*, Ellen?"

"I didn't say he was doing anything," I protested. "Please don't tell him that I said he was, because I didn't!" Then I began to shake as I silently recalled the probation session of more than four years ago; I knew I would face one again if I spoke now. Just having this conversation was jeopardizing the fragile lifeline I had reconnected to my therapist since my earlier "sin." "Please, Tony, we'll have to change the subject, or you'll have to go," I finally told him. He refused to do either.

He persisted in his questioning, as he sought to free me from my pain, and both of us from our illusions about Dr. Leonard. He spoke to my returning silence about the ethics of such a situation, the reasoning behind the rules of conduct that prohibited a psychiatrist from sleeping with a patient, and the terrible inequality of such encounters. That was when he first explained to me what Dr. Leonard himself had taught Tony about transference the day following the Christmas party in 1974.

"The occurrence of transference in a therapeutic relationship is part of why a sexual relationship with a patient is so unethical for the therapist, Ellen," he said, more pleading than explaining. He went on to explain that if I was seeking the approval from my doctor that I had needed to get from my parents, where was my agreement to participate in sexual encounters coming from—how I felt about the man, or my need for parental acceptance? If I had wanted the love of my parents and had transferred that need to be loved to my therapist—was my participation motivated by a romantic desire sparked and earned by the man himself, or by the implication that this was how I could finally earn that love? The possibilities for the strings that the therapist might pull in order to guarantee patient participation seemed endless for Tony. He listed many. Then he added that for a therapist to pull any one of them for the purpose of his own sexual gratification was "disgusting."

Tony talked like this for quite some time, urging me intermittently to talk about what had happened to me. But it was not until half the night had passed that he spoke the one line that made the difference to me. I had already stopped denying the existence of a sexual past with Dr. Leonard, but instead was arguing that "someday I will be able to understand it—someday when I am perfectly healthy."

"No, Ellen, you will never be able to understand it the way you think you will. You can't possibly, because it can't be understood."

With that, I felt a weight had been lifted off my shoulders. I felt no anger, no contempt, no vengeance. I only felt free. Slowly, in generalities, I began to tell Tony what he wanted to know. The details were unimportant; speaking about it *was*. The fury I saw in Tony's eyes directed toward Dr. Leonard was not important; seeing that Tony did not find Dr. Leonard's behavior rational or comprehensible *was*. Hearing that Dr. Leonard's actions might have been insane was not important; hearing that my reactions had not been, *was*.

Tony and I talked well into the night. We talked about what had happened to me, what he had learned that day, and what we would do next. We were sharing this experience in words,

147

but not in feeling. Tony was livid, enraged, and horrified as he listened to the bits and pieces I told him. I was feeling only relief.

In the days that followed that turning point, I prepared myself for the termination of my therapy. This time, it was my intellect that dictated my plan, not my emotions. I knew that I must leave therapy, but I still felt so tied to my therapist that all I could feel was panic over what he might do to me when I told him. Even at that point, I didn't hate him. I still only knew how to fear him.

It was during these days that I first understood how dependent my life was on Dr. Leonard. "But only Dr. Leonard can help me with my problems," I told Tony one evening.

"No, Ellen, that's what he wants you to believe. That's not how it really is," Tony replied.

But Dr. Leonard's words had been carved in stone; they still felt like my gospel.

Dr. Leonard had been on vacation during the time of my discussion with Tony. This not only gave me extra weeks to prepare and practice for the hour of action, as I had learned to do in the past in anticipation of confrontations with him over lesser issues, but it also afforded me time to talk to Linda. That was when I first learned of the full set of circumstances surrounding her own encounter with Dr. Leonard. Although there had not been sexual intercourse, a night in Dr. Leonard's bed at the beach house had been enough to cause Linda unspoken turmoil and pain for a long time. Now there were three of us, and I had to wonder how many more there were.

Once Tony had spoken with me and after I had spoken with Linda and, of course, Greg, the four of us spent many hours at my dining room table discussing the matter. Linda and I dwelled on our own pasts with Dr. Leonard, as well as on the story of Tony's friend, comparing notes and finding some comfort in the fact that our confusion and self-doubts had not been unique products of our own neurosis. Tony dwelled on his

148

shock and anger over what he considered to be a blatant violation of trust and professional conduct. This issue was far easier
for him to judge than the Christmas party had been; this time,
he wasn't the victim. And while Linda and I rummaged
through the history of our therapy, and while Tony tried in vain
to reconcile his adoration of Dr. Leonard with his new fallen
idol, Greg remained my only source of stability. He had not
been shocked by the information we had given him, only angered. He didn't have to deal with the contradictory images of
Dr. Leonard, as his brother and I did. Greg confided in us that
his biggest *problem* during the two years of his therapy had been
that he could never trust Dr. Leonard enough to tell him anything. Now he was learning that there was good cause for his
gut-level response to Dr. Leonard, and he was relieved at the
prospect of not having to face any more of Dr. Leonard's tirades
about how Greg's distrust of him indicated serious problems.

When I was alone, I spent my time rehearsing the words I
would say to Dr. Leonard upon the termination of my therapy,
and as I did so, I vacillated between tears of relief and fear of
confrontation. When I thought of that first night in his apartment, the wrestling in bed that I had never been able to comprehend and over which I had felt so inadequate, and his
judgments on me after, I could not wait to leave this man. But
when I recalled my probationary session, I trembled at the
thought of having to deal with his anger one more time in our
final meeting.

I wondered, would I be able to stand up to him? Would I be
able to answer his insinuations that my "faulty psychology" was
the real culprit? Would I be able to see through the tactics that
he used so often to make me believe that I was, once again,
being a "difficult patient"? Would I be able to resist if, then, he
offered me "one more chance"?

I wanted to be able to confront Dr. Leonard in person. Not
only did it seem like the proper and courageous thing to do, but
I thought that a face-to-face meeting would help me achieve the
termination of this nightmare. The thought of such a meeting,

however, threw me into such a panic that I sought out a crisis-intervention session from a new psychiatrist.

"A personal confrontation is the right way to handle this," I told the psychiatrist after I had filled him in on the story, "but I'm petrified."

"Right for whom?" he asked, after expressing outrage over what had been done to me. "You don't owe that bastard a thing, and you owe it to yourself to make this as easy on you as possible. My feeling is that you don't even owe him a phone call!"

I knew he was right, but terminating my relationship with Dr. Leonard was something I could not do without explanation. *That* I could not live with. But I would do it in the easiest way possible for me. I decided to handle it over the phone.

My next session was scheduled for the Monday afternoon of his return from vacation. I would phone him in the morning to cancel my session—and our relationship. I prepared myself for the worst possible reactions and rehearsed answers for all those possibilities. I made an outline of what I wanted to say, and underneath each heading, I wrote the briefest statement that would deliver the message I had in mind. I did not want a dialogue or debate on the matter. I only wanted him to know that I was leaving and to have an overall understanding as to the reason. With that in mind, and with my pad of paper in front of me, I picked up the receiver and, with sweaty palms and shortness of breath, dialed my therapist one last time.

"Hello," he answered. It was nearing ten o'clock and he sounded rushed to prepare for the day that would shortly begin.

I gulped. "Dr. Leonard, this is Ellen."

The sternness and tension in my voice must have gone undetected by Dr. Leonard, as did the difficulty in my breathing, as he responded with a friendly casualness. "Hi, Ellen. I'm busy right now. May I call you back during lunch?"

Already my script had to be abandoned. I had not prepared for a delay. "There's no need to call me back, Dr. Leonard. I'm calling to terminate therapy with you, so you can cancel my session for the day."

I waited for him to yell at me, to call me names, or to pass judgment on me. He did none of these things. His tone of voice shifted from friendly familiarity to quiet and cautious reservation. He sounded almost shy as he responded, "In that case, Ellen, I'll make time to talk to you now. What's going on?"

"I'm terminating therapy for two reasons, Dr. Leonard. The first is the sexual relationship that you instigated and promoted during the course of my therapy, and all of the confusion and pain it caused me.

"The second reason is that you used your position as my therapist to *diagnose away* all of that pain as symptomatic of an unhealthy psychology, while passing judgment on me for being unable to cope with your abuse. My probation session is the best example of that. For that session alone, I should have left you a long time ago."

He paused, and then answered only, "I understand." Then, with an emphasized politeness and noticable nervousness to his voice, he asked me to walk over to his apartment so that we might discuss this in person. "I'll even cancel my morning appointments," he offered.

"No, Dr. Leonard, I do not want to see you," I answered as I felt my strength growing.

"I understand," he repeated. "Could you tell me, at least, what triggered this decision?"

"No, I can't," I answered, and I did not tell him why I could not. Tony had made me promise to leave that part of it to him for his upcoming session with Dr. Leonard the following day. He wanted Dr. Leonard to have no advance warning of his knowledge on the subject, and I had agreed to let him have his element of surprise.

"Please, Ellen," he begged, "can't I get you to come talk to me in person about this?"

"No, Dr. Leonard. There is nothing else I want to discuss with you."

Then there was a long, long silence. I thought for a moment that he might have put the phone down and walked away, just to have the satisfaction of leaving me on hold at the other end. I considered hanging up when he finally broke the silence.

Slowly, deliberately, thoughtfully, and softly, he said, "I've suspected for a long time that what I have done to you has damaged you."

I was stunned! I was not prepared at all for such a remark—for such a confession. I picked up the pen that lay by the pad of paper and wrote down his words in the silence that followed:

I've suspected for a long time that what I have done to you has damaged you.

I knew I would want to review these words later.

Now he was speaking again. "Could I come to your apartment if you don't want to make the trip over here? I really would like to talk to you about this."

With more strength than I thought myself capable of, with more courage than I had experienced during any point prior to this one, I said firmly: "Dr. Leonard, I can't count how many times during the last five years I have begged you to talk about this very subject. Each time I did, you either refused to discuss it, or you intimated a serious neurosis because of my need to discuss it. Now it's you who wants to talk about it, and I'm just not interested in discussing it with you anymore. There's nothing in it for me at this point; you're no longer my doctor." I paused, and then added, "Let me put it this way, Dr. Leonard: *The trade is over.*"

"I understand," he said once more, this time with regret. He seemed to.

In a tone of resignation, he said, "I hope that when you get done weighing all the benefits of therapy against the damage I have done to you, that the benefits will come out ahead."

"That kind of determination takes time, Dr. Leonard. Right now, I can only see the harm," I replied.

"I understand," he said for the last time.

"If you do, then there's no more to be said—except good-bye."

"Good-bye, Ellen," he returned. "I really mean it when I say that I wish you the best of luck."

I hung up the phone and it was over. Five and a half years of living for my therapist's approval, five and a half years of struggling toward some elusive standard of mental health and femininity, five and a half years of seeking his guidance and support—it was all over. Everything around which my life had seemed to revolve for all those years had come to an abrupt end, and I found myself floundering in a pool of depression, searching for a new direction, a new lifeline.

I tried hard to feel some anger toward my former therapist. I could not. Intellectually, I had only just begun to understand what he had done to me. But emotionally, all I could feel was relief at not having to please him, at not having to fear him, at not having to struggle to feel what he thought I should feel but could not. But anger? No, I felt no anger, no resentment, no bitterness. Not yet, anyway.

I wondered whether I could survive without his direction, his orders, his guidelines, his rules. I even wondered if I would miss seeing him every other week. I recalled, once again, his frequent reminder that no one could help me except him, and again, I wondered if it might not be true. Had I rid myself of a devil in control of my life, or the last hope for my salvation? Had he been a deterrent to my happiness, or the last remaining key to it? Perhaps, I reasoned, it was necessary to get this much worse in therapy before I could get any better. Only one thing seemed clear: that I could not yet *feel* for sure what I had only begun to understand in principle.

I thought about where I would go. I had come to New York to do therapy with Dr. Leonard. Now there was nothing holding me in the city. I was free to go wherever I liked. I knew Greg disliked Manhattan as much as I. Surely, he would go with me.

Questions whirled through my head like a cyclone. I questioned everything from who I really was to where I should be living. Now I was on my own to find the answers, and I felt lost and scared and depressed. I could not know, however, that as desperate and depressed as I was during the week following my conversation with Dr. Leonard, things were to get worse—much worse—before they would ever get better.

12

TAKING ◇ SIDES

Summer 1977

Within a day of my terminating therapy with Dr. Leonard, he was announcing to his remaining patients his intent to take an "indefinite sabbatical" beginning in August of 1977, just three months away. The bewilderment this caused for many of them was easy for me to understand. It was even easier for me to comprehend the sense of fright and desertion this evoked, as I knew that that was how I would have responded to such news only a short time ago. Word of Dr. Leonard's sabbatical spread quickly, as did the reason he was offering for it. "He's tired," these patients explained. "He says he needs a long rest. He says that no one can do the intense kind of therapy he does without eventually burning out."

To his other patients (besides Greg and Linda) whom I considered among my friends, I revealed the issue which had for so long been a guarded secret. I wanted to explain the circumstances that had preceded Dr. Leonard's announcement of needed rest, partly because I felt this information might prompt them to leave their therapy sooner than the date of Dr. Leonard's own choosing. Surely, they would see the issues as Tony had, for they were not blinded and confused by the same muddle that I, a victim, had been. They were capable of being objective and acting accordingly.

I also sought out my friends for reassurance. Feeling disoriented and alone, I needed to cling to anything in my life that was stable. Eric's presence and needs forced me to maintain control, and Greg's support and comfort were endless and sincere, but they were not enough for this dazed and frightened woman. I had lost my parents. I had lost Dr. Leonard. Now I desperately needed my friends. I turned to them for reinforcement of what was good in my life, and more importantly, for a test of reality: was happiness—was life itself—possible after judging and leaving Dr. Leonard? I needed an affirmative answer to my unspoken question, but the reaction of the first friend I approached with my story forewarned what was to happen with many of those friends on whom I had been counting.

Robert Berger and I had known each other ever since my days in Chicago. He had been one of those who had "boycotted" my marriage to David. But since that time, we had become friends—he, forgiving my marriage and I, forgiving his extremism. A Ph.D. working as a research scientist at a prestigious university, he was one of my more accomplished friends. We saw each other often, usually when he commuted into New York from out of town for his sessions with Dr. Leonard. He loved me as a friend, and told me so often. I felt no fear in approaching Robert with this information. Not only did I believe a man of his ability would have no problem with this issue, but he had told me once how a former therapist of his live-in girlfriend had tried to seduce her. He had been appalled that therapists did such things, while I had remained silent in response to his expression of horror. Further, his professed care for me told me that I could expect his support and warmth in my time of need.

I was mistaken.

I called Robert and told him of the recent events. He heard what I had to say, responded with stunned sympathy, and then, after having time to think about it, answered my long-distance phone communication by mail.[1]

He began his letter by saying that he was writing because of what our friendship *used to* mean to him. I prepared myself for what was to follow.

He could not disprove what I had told him, he said, nor would he even try. Instead, he would reach his conclusion that Dr. Leonard was guiltless of any improper conduct with me by relying on the information he already had. That information was everything he knew about Dr. Leonard first hand, and Robert's understanding that "contradictions do not exist." The latter was meant to refer to that part of Objectivism which teaches that contradictions do not exist in reality—in *metaphysical* reality. In other words, a grain of sand or a bead of water has a particular nature unto itself, and cannot, therefore, take on attributes that are contrary to its nature. It cannot be what it is and be what it is not, all at the same time. Ergo, "contradictions do not exist."

Robert had taken this axiom and extended its meaning into the realm of human psychology, a realm it does not legitimately claim. He explained his leap from the metaphysical to the psychological as he continued his letter. He said that Dr. Leonard was the finest man he had ever known, as well as the best psychiatrist in the world, and that what I had said about Dr. Leonard contradicted those facts. Since contradictions don't exist, Robert explained, Dr. Leonard could not possibly be guilty of any impropriety. Robert said that he not only knew Dr. Leonard was innocent of any misconduct, he also claimed that he knew Dr. Leonard's actions with me were ethical and honorable, and essential for productive therapy. He hoped that I would see the error of my ways, but told me, regardless, to "go to hell." He signed it simply: Robert Berger.

[1]Permission to reproduce this letter verbatim was requested from its writer, the person herein called Robert Berger. Through a letter from his lawyer, permission was denied.

The letter not only braced me for the responses I would continue to receive from other friends, it told me that blind devotion to Dr. Leonard had not been a unique phenomenon for me. I was discovering that I had no monopoly on having been duped by this therapist for so many years. What was so hard to understand was *how* it happened, *why* it happened, that so many people gave so much allegiance for so many years to one man such as him. Was its root in Objectivism? Was there something in between the lines of the philosophy that both taught independent thinking and proper reasoning, and dictated a result resembling the cults of religious leaders? Or was it something in the black and white print that went undetected by so many intelligent readers? Perhaps it was not in the philosophy, at all. Perhaps it was a coincidence, a fluke, that Dr. Leonard and all of his loyal patients were students of Objectivism. Was it, then, a charisma about the man that led to such blind worship of him? Was there some special skill he had that made so many people either twist or ignore all that they professed to have learned from their philosophy?

I received only one other letter similar to Robert's. It came from Robert's girlfriend. But I received innumerable phone calls, from men and women alike, who *condemned* me for terminating my own therapy and for the reason they had learned was behind my doing so. In one call, I was accused of "destroying the closest thing Man has ever had to a god." In another, I was threatened with retaliation for causing the closing of Dr. Leonard's practice. The connection between Dr. Leonard's sabbatical and the termination of my therapy had been made, and I was being blamed for the downfall of a hero.

It was during these days and weeks of seeking answers, talking to friends and losing them, and screening the threatening phone calls from the harmless ones, that I came upon the pad of paper on which I had written Dr. Leonard's words:

I've suspected for a long time that what I have done to you has damaged you.

I read the words over and over, trying to grasp what it was I thought I was seeing in them. Something had gnawed away at me ever since I had heard those words and I searched for the source of my uneasiness. Then, like a flash in the darkness, I saw what had been too painful to recognize in that phrase before: he knew he had been harming me, but that did not stop him from continuing to do so.

It had seemed a slightly easier injury to live with when I could believe that he cared for me too much to knowingly do me harm. It had been a different matter when I thought he was simply misguided, mistaken, or even deranged. I could have been more content with the past, thinking his intentions had been only the best, albeit erroneous. But I could not handle what I was understanding now.

I wanted to rush to his apartment, throw open the door and demand an explanation. "What do you mean, *you suspected for a long time?*" I wanted to ask. "How long is *long?* How long were you screwing me and suspecting that it was damaging me?"

I wished in that moment that I was a scientist so that I could ask him contemptuously, as one colleague to another, "What did you do with your suspicions, *Doctor?* Did you analyze them, draw a diagnosis, and try to find a cure for the wounds you inflicted? Or did you just shrug your shoulders in a lack of concern before pulling down your pants just one more time?"

I thought of all the things I wished I could say to him now. I wished I had been sharp enough to see this meaning in his words at the time he had said them. Then I cried over the realization that I had not mattered to him at all, not as a person, and certainly not as a patient. I knew I had been used, and for the first time since Tony had come to my apartment that evening in May, I was angry.

When word had traveled through the grapevine that I had terminated my therapy because of sexual encounters with Dr. Leonard, some patients questioned their therapist about these "rumors," while others just laughed it off, hypothesizing that I must have learned about other encounters he had had and was

159

feeling like "the woman scorned." Most were satisfied with the explanation he provided, and they remained in therapy until the date of his sabbatical. It was sometime in June when I first heard what that explanation was.

"Dr. Leonard said that it was part of your therapy and that you gave your consent to have such therapy with him. He said that you signed a consent form giving him permission to do what he did with you," one acquaintance told me over the phone. She, too, had called to condemn my actions, but was eager for me to know that she had sought both sides to the story. This second-hand account of Dr. Leonard's explanation was not the only one I would hear. And when I had heard it for the fifth time, my growing anger sought a form of ventilation. I quickly recalled how he had stood before me, so self-righteously, so indignantly, and proclaimed, while pointing to his bedroom, that that was one thing and therapy was another. I remembered how many times I had begged him for an explanation, only to be answered with impatience, aggravation, innuendo, or silence. I thought about all the sessions where my anxiety and pain would not be addressed because "our sex has nothing to do with what goes on in here." And I knew, without any doubt or reservation, that I would take him to court.

The first person I told of my decision was Linda, and I urged her to consider doing the same. Linda, however, was leery of the publicity that such a case might bring, and she needed more time to weigh her fear of that possibility against her desire to act against Dr. Leonard. Within weeks, the latter won out.

Then I thought of the story with which Tony had come to me the month before. I thought of the woman whose story it had been, and I telephoned her to tell her of my decision to sue Dr. Leonard for malpractice. I hoped that she would join me in the action, but her agreement would have no bearing on my determination to follow through with my own decision, just as Linda's had not. Perhaps, I thought, she will be just as anxious to make a statement about this as I am. And I was not so naïve as to not know that a corroborating story could not hurt. After all, Dr. Leonard had never penetrated Linda, and Tony's friend was the only woman I knew of, besides myself, whom he had.

I had only met Patricia Osborne at infrequent parties or gatherings. I had spoken with her in casual conversation on these occasions and it had been quite some time since the last time we had seen each other. We had never become close friends, but that did not make me uncomfortable now that I was contemplating approaching her with such a delicate topic. I had always liked Patti whenever we had been together. I had found her to be friendly, outgoing, and warm, and I remembered her as a woman who smiled a lot and laughed easily. I did not worry about contacting her now, under these circumstances. I looked forward to it.

"I'd rather castrate him," she said, not in jest, "but a malpractice suit sounds good for a second choice." She agreed to join me, so long as I would do all the leg work in finding us a lawyer.

We spoke at great length during this conversation, as we compared our experiences and found comfort in knowing we were each not alone. It was also during this talk that she told me she had had to seek additional therapy after leaving Dr. Leonard, "to try and put the pieces back together again." She had seen Dr. Blumenthal for that therapy.

"Dr. Blumenthal?" I asked.

"Yes," she told me. "Apparently, he had already treated other victims of Dr. Leonard before I went to see him."

I was flabbergasted at what I was hearing. First, I was learning that there had been other women besides Linda, Patti, and me. I had strongly suspected as much, but my suspicions had been strictly circumstantial deductions. Second, I now had to wonder whether Dr. Blumenthal might have indeed known "exactly" what I was talking about when I had telephoned him for help four and a half years earlier. He had said that he did, but I had always believed that we were each referring to a different matter. We *had* to be. Had he truly known, he certainly

---

161

would have helped me. Especially since he referred me to Dr. Leonard. Refusal to help under such circumstances would have been so outrageous, I could not have even considered the possibility.

Patti's treatment under Dr. Blumenthal did not commence until some years after my telephone conversation with him, but her reference to his treatment of other victims *before* that, led me to reconsider whether Dr. Blumenthal's declaration of knowledge might have been accurate. In light of his own words to me then, it was hard to doubt that conclusion now. But without more information on Dr. Blumenthal's state of knowledge at the time of our conversation, I could not be sure.

What I did know for sure, however, was that Dr. Blumenthal had knowledge of Dr. Leonard's abusive conduct *now* and had had that knowledge for some time. Dr. Blumenthal had never, however, called me back to withdraw his high recommmendation of Dr. Leonard or his refusal to help me. I was furious at what I saw as gross cowardice, and I told Patti so.

"He did stop recommending Dr. Leonard, Ellen," she explained in his defense.

"For God's sake, Patti, I learned that Dr. Blumenthal was no longer recommending Dr. Leonard *from Dr. Leonard*. He said it was due to an ideological disagreement! So what the hell did it mean that he 'stopped recommending Dr. Leonard'? Was that his way of taking a stand? Of helping the women he had already referred? Of correcting the error he had made in his recommendation?"

Patti, however, was less interested in pursuing a discussion on Dr. Blumenthal than she was in expressing her long-suppressed feelings about Dr. Leonard. We returned to our original topic.

"I thought about suing him before," she told me, "but I was too afraid that no one would believe me. So I just left therapy and kept my mouth shut."

Then she thanked me for coming forward and saying out loud what he had done. Now she was free to speak after such a long period of silence. Perhaps others would be, as well.

The issue had been joined. There were few, if any, of Dr. Leonard's patients who did not know what I was accusing him of. The line had been drawn and sides had been taken. He lost many patients. I lost many friends. I was, however, able to take solace in the fact that, for the time being, he would stop practicing his particular style of psychotherapy.

I had ended my phone conversation with Patti with a promise to contact her just as soon as a lawyer could be found to handle our cases. That would prove to be more difficult than I ever expected.

13

THE ◇ LAWYERS

Adam Rosenberg maintained a legal practice in Hicksville, Long Island, as well as in Miami, Florida. At least that is what his business card said. I had retained him to handle my divorce at an earlier date, and now I was seeking his help on a more complicated matter.

"I don't know if this is the kind of thing you handle, but you're the only lawyer I know in New York."

He was curious about the situation I had briefly described to him over the phone and invited Linda and me in for further discussion. Once in his office, he asked many questions about what had transpired between Dr. Leonard and me. And he wanted it in detail.

I buried my embarrassment and answered him as directly as I could, reliving almost every moment of sexual contact with Dr. Leonard. Then he questioned me about my family background, my personal life, my sex life besides Dr. Leonard, my past romantic relationships, and "whatever horrible facts" I could think of that I "would never want anyone to know." He explained that this was all necessary information for his final decision on whether or not to take the case.

I answered obligingly, as I needed a decision immediately.

"Dr. Leonard is going on sabbatical in less than two months," I told him, "and I have reason to believe that he will be leaving the state. He's supposed to be moving to Florida, but I don't know where."

He agreed that time was of the essence, and agreed to take the case. Next, he brought up the issue of money.

"I only have five hundred dollars in my savings account," I told him. Linda echoed my response. "Will that be enough to start?" I asked, adding that Patti's five hundred would be following shortly.

He agreed to take the fifteen hundred dollars plus a one-third percentage of whatever the suit might bring. I wrote him out a check for the entirety of my account and left.

After a week's passing, Mr. Rosenberg notified me that he had written a letter to Dr. Leonard's insurance company.

"A letter? To his insurance company? Why?" I wanted to know.

He explained that he needed to determine where the malpractice insurance carrier stood on the matter.

When another week had passed, he telephoned to say that he had received a very unsatisfactory response from the insurance company, and that the matter would have to be pursued through other channels. He would contact me when he had more information. I did not understand his method. I wanted to sue Dr. Leonard, not an insurance company. I wanted to see Dr. Leonard put in a position of having to give answers to questions. I wanted to see him exposed for what he really was. I did not understand this insurance company business, but then I was not a lawyer.

More time passed, and no word came from our lawyer. Worrying about time running out before Dr. Leonard left for unknown places, I phoned Mr. Rosenberg for an update only to be told by a secretary that Mr. Rosenberg was "out" and would return my call when he could.

Days passed, and still no return phone call from my lawyer. I phoned his office again, and again I heard that he was "out" but would return my call when he could. This sequence recurred several more times, until one day, when I phoned his office after five o'clock, Mr. Rosenberg himself answered the telephone.

He seemed annoyed with my calling him after business hours. He seemed equally annoyed when he made reference to the pile of message slips with my name on it.

"Mr. Rosenberg, I need to know what is happening. Dr. Leonard is leaving town in less than four weeks and I don't know what you've done—if anything."

"I am pressed on another matter right now, Ellen. You'll have to be patient." He talked about having a large sum of money wrapped up in a movie theater business, and the movies for the season had to be "bid on," I think he said. I didn't pay much attention to the details of his private business deals. I only wanted to know what he was doing for me.

He assured me, contradicting his words of our first meeting, that the time element was not a real problem in my case. Dr. Leonard could always be found in Florida if papers were not served prior to his departure. I was, he said, not to worry.

But I did worry. I worried about whether he was the lawyer to handle this case. I phoned him back immediately and asked for an appointment to see him the following day. He agreed.

I had never fired a lawyer before, but my apprehension over the prospect was mildly reminiscent of what firing my therapist had been. Linda and I made the long trip from Manhattan to Hicksville together, and I carefully selected the words I would use, and tried them out on my friend for approval. I promised myself that I would not show my anger nor lose my control with this man; that might interfere with the message I wanted to deliver, as well as the refunding of our money on which I planned to insist.

"Before you say anything," he began before I had barely made myself comfortable, "I think I should tell you that I have to withdraw from your case. I just don't have the time to handle it properly."

I relaxed. He had handled the matter for me and we could part amicably. "I'm glad you see that," I said with relief, "because that was the conclusion we had reached, as well." Then I asked him for a refund of the retainer which we had paid him.

"But I've done work on the case," he answered incredulously. "I think I'm entitled to be paid for my services."

I was astounded by his refusal to refund the retainer we had paid him, but not nearly as astounded as by his proclamation of work done. "What have you done?" I implored.

"I wrote the letter to the insurance company," he replied in his defense.

"But we didn't pay you a thousand dollars to write a letter!" Patti had not yet mailed him her five-hundred-dollar payment. "Further, we paid you to handle an entire case, not a piece of it," I retorted.

"That might be," he answered, "but I do not return retainers when I have been dismissed from a case. The fee is always forfeited in such cases."

Dismissed? He had withdrawn before I could dismiss him. "I thought we *both* agreed that you could not handle this case," I argued.

"I don't want to argue over this," he said. "I am willing to compromise. I will return half of the money—but no more than that."

I was not up to arguing, either. My mind was preoccupied with Dr. Leonard's impending departure, as well as deciding on my next course of action. I felt grateful that Patti had been so delinquent in sending Mr. Rosenberg her money, thus reducing our total loss. I asked him on the spot for the fifty percent of what Linda and I had paid him, explaining that we would need it to hire another attorney. He wrote out a check, complaining while doing so that he was taking it out of his personal account, as he could not justify the withdrawal from the firm's own books. I accepted our check and left in a panic. With less than four weeks before Dr. Leonard's sabbatical, we still had no law-yer.

After I had hired Mr. Rosenberg, I had started researching and reading everything I could on the subject of psychiatric mal-practice. One book in particular was informative and encourag-ing. The book jacket stated that the book's author was a practicing attorney in New York City. I looked up the name *Marvin T. Stern*, and phoned for an appointment.

A friendly and distinguished-looking man, Mr. Stern tried to put me at ease before commencing with his questions. He, too, wanted details on what had happened, but his professional demeanor quickly disappeared upon hearing the answers.

"Then the encounters moved to fellatio," I was explaining.

"To what?" he asked in surprise.

"Fellatio."

"Fellatio?" he asked.

"Yes."

"When you say 'fellatio,' what exactly do you mean?"

"What do you mean, what do I mean?" I did not understand what the problem was.

"What exactly did you do?" he asked.

"He told me to suck on his penis, so I did what he told me to do."

"You put his penis into your mouth?!" He appeared stunned. Shocked. In a state of disbelief and wonderment, all at once. I could not tell if it was the act itself that surprised him, or that such a thing had occurred between a doctor and patient. I did not question him to find out which.

"Yes, I put his penis into my mouth. That is generally how fellatio occurs, is it not?" I was not trying to be smart with him, I was trying to lighten the mood that had just fallen on the room.

The conversation continued like this for well over an hour. At the conclusion, he agreed to take the case and asked for a retainer of whatever we could afford, recognizing that it wasn't going to be much. He was very understanding of our limited resources.

"When can I expect to hear from you?" I asked before leaving.

He explained that he was not a trial lawyer, and that one would have to be chosen before we could move on the case at all. In response, I explained to him the time crunch and he agreed that he would need to move swiftly.

Weeks passed, and the only word that came from Mr. Stern was that no trial lawyer could be found. With only a little more than one week remaining before Dr. Leonard's departure, I phoned my new lawyer to either get the name of a trial lawyer or to dismiss him from the case. I did the latter, as he still had not found a trial lawyer.

Initially, he, too, refused to refund the retainer we had paid him. We both became angry on the phone and he rudely said good-bye to me before hanging up. But before the desperation of my situation even had a chance to sink in, Mr. Stern was calling back to apologize. Remembering the unfortunate experience we had had with Mr. Rosenberg, he wanted us to have whatever money we had paid him so that we might hire another attorney. Then he stated his regret over his inability to help us in this case. He thought the case to be an important one, and wished us well in it. We parted on good terms.

There was one week left before Dr. Leonard's rumored date of departure and we had no lawyer. I reached in my purse and withdrew a folded and worn sheet of paper which I had received from the American Bar Association. Sometime during my early doubts over Mr. Rosenberg's competence, I had phoned the ABA asking for a recommendation of a lawyer specializing in malpractice cases. They could not give me one name, but promised to mail me a list from which I could make my own selection. The list arrived after retaining Mr. Stern. Now I was scanning the names with which the organization had provided me.

"Take a pin, close your eyes, and pick one," Linda advised me. *Fuchsberg & Fuchsberg* won the pick.

Abraham Fuchsberg was the half of Fuchsberg & Fuchsberg I was to see, the voice on the other end of the phone told me. I was not told, however, that four other gentlemen would be privy to our meeting; but that was what awaited us when Linda and I entered Mr. Fuchsberg's office. It was Mr. Fuchsberg, however, who was clearly in charge. He invited us to sit down, introduced the other men who were already present, issued an order for the appearance of another attorney who had not yet arrived, and began the conference.

Mr. Fuchsberg explained that all but one of the men present were attorneys with his firm. The exception was, I believe he said, a state senator, and he asked our permission for this man to remain, assuring us that confidentiality was understood by all those present. Four men, five men, or twenty men, it did not matter. One less would not have been any less intimidating than what I was facing now. We agreed to let the senator stay.

Mr. Fuchsberg began the questioning. He did it with the utmost diplomacy and professionalism. He did not request to hear unnecessary details. He did not ask for "horrible facts," and chuckled when I asked if he wanted to hear them. He did not gasp at what details I did give him in response to his questions, nor did he show any sympathy or sign of understanding. He simply asked what was important and did not dwell on any sordid details that might elaborate the point.

He opened the floor to the other attorneys and they were all equally objective, professional, and courteous in their questioning. Only once did I receive any indication at all of what any of them was feeling. Following my answer to one of Mr. Fuchsberg's later questions, one attorney remarked, "I'm having a strong visceral response." When I asked what he meant, someone else replied, "He's going to be sick."

When all the questioning was completed, I explained to Mr. Fuchsberg what I had explained to the two attorneys preceding him: time was of the essence. I asked him how soon he could begin to act on the case. Much to my surprise, he responded by stating that no decision had yet been made to take the case. Given the time element, however, he would not ask me to wait until the following day for an answer. He asked us to return to the waiting room while he conferred with his colleagues. Shortly thereafter, we were invited back into the office where, for the first time, I saw Mr. Fuchsberg smiling. I had a lawyer.

"Where does Dr. Leonard live?" he was asking me now.

"In Peter Cooper Village, at 360 First Avenue," I answered.

"Don't we have someone in the office that lives over there?" he was asking his staff. It was determined that there was such a person in the firm, and he was beckoned to Mr. Fuchsberg's office. After he spoke to the man, Mr. Fuchsberg turned to speak to me. "Dr. Leonard will be served before dinnertime tonight."

"What time?" I asked, still not believing that things could actually get done so quickly.

He thought a moment and replied, "Before seven."

Remembering Dr. Leonard's work schedule, I was pleased that he would still have patients in his apartment when the papers were served. It seemed just that he would.

Now the discussion turned to money. Very casually, Mr. Fuchsberg stated that his firm required a retainer of fifteen hundred dollars *per case*.

My heart sank as I saw the wheels of justice, which had just begun to turn, come to a screeching halt. "All I have left is two hundred and fifty dollars, but I could pay you the rest over time." Linda echoed my reply.

Without missing a beat, Mr. Fuchsberg replied that he did not wish to leave us without a savings account. He told us to pay whatever we could and that that would be sufficient. Time payments would not be necessary. He asked us to pass the same message on to Patti, and then explained what the previous two lawyers had explained about taking a third percentage of whatever the case brought. I did not want to ask him, What if we lose?

It could not have been more than a few weeks since I had retained Mr. Fuchsberg, when I opened the Sunday edition of *The New York Times* and found Dr. Lonnie Franklin Leonard's name, along with Linda's, Patti's, and mine, in an article explaining the news that a reporter had uncovered when papers had been filed with the court. By the end of that week, the *Daily News* was carrying a similar story, and local networks were broadcasting it to the city. And much to my dismay, the *National Enquirer* also ran the story. They even sent a reporter to my apartment who stood on the other side of the door I had closed in his face after discovering he was a reporter, asking me questions like, "Are you and Linda lesbian lovers?" After getting no response, he slipped a business card under the door, just in case I changed my mind about being interviewed, and left.

It was through the New York papers, though, that I learned how much I was suing Dr. Leonard for: *four million dollars per complainant,* the paper said.

I phoned my lawyer, disturbed that I had not been consulted on nor informed of this decision. I also questioned the sanity of a man who would ask for such a large amount. Mr. Fuchsberg explained to me then that the amount being sought is more of a statement on the abhorrence of Dr. Leonard's actions, not the amount that can be expected in award. There was no need to consult me, he said, because I could not have determined the magnitude of the case from the perspective of a legal issue. I was reassured, and my mind was set free to deal with the phone calls to my apartment, which the articles had produced.

With the exception of a few reporters, all of the calls were coming from former patients of Dr. Leonard. All but one of them were women. And all the women had, at one time or another, been victims of the same treatment. Some called anonymously; others were willing to give their name and wanting to help in any way they could. Some wanted to file their own suit against Dr. Leonard. Some just wanted to go on record as willing to testify. And some said they just wanted to say "thank you" for being able to do what they could not.

Some of the calls were particularly painful for me, as the voice on the other end "just wanted to talk about what Dr. Leonard had done to [her]," because she had never told it to anyone before. Some would not reveal their identities before they spoke, but cried into the phone as if we were old friends. Others told me who they were, and I recalled meeting some of them years ago at a party or in Dr. Leonard's waiting room.

I listened to their stories and I cried with them and for them in a way I had yet to do for myself. Besides needing to talk, most of the callers needed to know *when* the sexual activity had occurred between Dr. Leonard and me. Was he sleeping with other women when he had been sleeping with them, they wanted to know, as they still held onto that last vestige of hope that they had been special to him.

When the dust had settled and the calls became less frequent, Mr. Fuchsberg was left with a list of five clients who were willing to file suit against Dr. Leonard and who he was willing to handle. And we were all left with a list of names of prospective witnesses and known victims.

It was when four of the five plaintiffs gathered for a meeting in Mr. Fuchsberg's office that I first met Nell. During a private dinner afterward, a small piece to the puzzle of my past with Dr. Leonard fell into place. We were sitting over drinks, telling each of our stories to the other, when I reached the point in my chronology with him concerning the open cosmetic bag in his bedroom. I told Nell how Dr. Leonard had maintained that he had already told me about "another woman" in his life, and I repeated to her now what he had been certain then had occurred in that discussion.

Her eyes widened as I spoke. With each detail of the conversation he had told me we had had, the amazement on her face grew more intense. When I finished, she looked directly at me and simply said: "That was me."

"What was you?" I asked.

"That was me he had that conversation with. Almost word

173

for word. He had that exact conversation with me—not you. Me!"

We continued our discussion, making note of his confused memory about what he was doing and saying to whom, but not dwelling on it. We did not know yet how significant that confusion actually was. We were to find out.

14

THE ◇ DEFENSE

The legal process had been set into motion, and all there was to do now was wait. Mr. Fuchsberg had estimated a two-year span between the time of filing our suits and the date that would be set for trial. He could not have known that his calculations would be short by over three years.

I left New York in the middle of 1978, almost one year after my first visit to a lawyer's office, but not before the loss of two more friends: Tony and Linda. It was in the middle weeks of autumn that Greg received a phone call at his office from Tony, stating that he no longer wished to be my friend. Greg was instructed by his brother to relay this message to me, with further instructions that I should not attempt to contact him for a discussion of the matter. No reasons were given for his decision, and when Greg asked for an explanation, Tony refused it.

Knowing what this would do to my already depressed state of mind, Greg reluctantly relayed Tony's words to me that night. And predictably, this new confusion, this new loss, devastated me. I did little else than cry for nearly two weeks, as I reviewed the details of all my latest encounters with Tony, looking for the moment of my error, the time of my offense—anything that might have caused my good friend to desert me.

It was not, I knew, an issue of Tony switching sides in the matter of Dr. Leonard. Tony had previously offered to help in our cases and had reiterated that position to Greg on the phone. So it was obviously a personal issue between Tony and me. But what, I wondered, had I done that was so horrible that I did not even deserve an explanation? I replayed every conversation that Tony and I had recently had, searching for the answer. I found none.

The strain under which Tony's relationship with Greg was placed as a result of Tony's abrupt discharge of me from his life, was exacerbated to the point of severing the closeness once shared by these two brothers. Tony met with Greg several weeks following the telephone conversation which had initiated Tony's message to me. It was during this meeting that Tony expressed his desire to keep their relationship unaffected by the change in the status of his relationship with me. So long as Greg understood that Tony would never want to see me or hear about me, their relationship could proceed as usual. But whereas Tony saw this as the means to maintaining the closeness he shared with his brother, Greg saw this as an emotional impossibility. It was like being asked to pretend that I didn't exist for him. His rejection of Tony's offer left a clear conclusion: the brothers would no longer speak.

Greg and I searched for possible explanations to Tony's bizarre and cruel behavior. But just as I alone had found no answers in this avenue of exploration, neither did we find any together.

"I think," Greg finally concluded, "that you are the baby that got thrown out with the bathwater."

I understood immediately what he was saying, and it was the most probable explanation I had heard so far. Tony's reaction to the discovery of Dr. Leonard's abuse had been one of total and absolute disgust and rejection. With anger, disappointment, and renewed conviction to a fundamental distrust of his fellow man, Tony had handled the destruction of his idol with a unilateral dismissal of everything in his life that was somehow connected to the therapist and Objectivism. He rejected Dr. Leonard, the entirety of his therapy, the former friends who sided with Dr. Leonard, the other friends and associations he had made through Objectivism—and me. It would be four years before Greg and I would learn that his hypothesis had been right. Until that time, Greg was silently shattered over his loss while I mourned the loss more openly.

Soon after my relationship with Tony had ended, my friendship with Linda began to sour. Again, without explanation, without reason, she began to call less and less frequently, and those times that she did were not of the same quality as they had once been. She no longer visited for long talks and leisurely dinners, or initiated evenings out at the movies or restaurants. And she seemed always to find excuses for turning down such invitations or suggestions from me.

Because Linda and I had always been able to talk out our differences in the past, I did not immediately conclude that her coolness toward me was the result of her changing feelings about our relationship. I assumed that she was going through a difficult time for reasons unrelated to me, and that she would discuss her problem when she felt ready.

"Give her space to work it through," Greg advised me. "She'll come to you when she's ready to talk about it."

His words told me what I already knew to be true: Linda would not do to me what Tony had done. After all, she had been just as puzzled and dismayed by Tony's treatment of me as I had been. To follow suit would not have been her way. But by Christmas of that year, 1977, we were proved wrong.

It was Christmas day when Linda phoned to ask if she could walk over to give Greg and me our Christmas present. I was elated over the implication that she wanted to spend time with us on the holiday, and joyfully agreed to have her visit. I did not question this change of attitude, I only welcomed it.

The look on her face as she walked through my front door told me that I had rejoiced too soon. This was not the face of a

177

friend who had come in love and warmth, bearing gifts and greetings for the season. This was the face of restrained hostility.

She took a seat at the dining room table, and waited for Greg and me to be seated across from her before she spoke.

"Here," she said in a huff, sliding a brown paper bag across the table. "Merry Christmas." She may as well have said "I hate you both," for that was the tone of her words.

Inside the brown paper bag was an unwrapped glass candle holder, the kind which holds water and oil, not sticks. The sticker bearing the hardware store's name was still stuck to the merchandise, with the price clearly marked below.

It was an awkward moment that followed. I did not know whether to thank her for the gift, or whether to seize this opportunity to ask her what the hell was wrong. She was delivering conflicting messages, and I did not know which one to address. In case I was misinterpreting the unspoken one, I decided to thank her for the thought and the gift. Greg did the same.

Before the uneasiness grew, Linda rose and announced she had intended to stay for only a minute. After a futile attempt to convince her to stay, she departed. That was the last time we ever spoke or met socially.

This time, I did not cry at the loss of a friend or in bewilderment. After all my losses, there was nothing left but the defense of callousness. Were it not for Greg's support and witness to this unintelligible behavior, I would have felt totally abandoned and confused. That I felt numb was a blessing.

There seemed to be no reason for waiting out the slow process of the legal system in a city that carried so many painful memories, so Greg and I returned to the Midwest, from where each of us had come, taking my son back to the place of his birth. At least there I had my grandmother and a sister who had recently reestablished a relationship with me. There I awaited notice of the next major step in my case against Lonnie Leonard: his examination before trial. During his deposition, he would be questioned extensively by my lawyers, just as I would be on a later date by his.

Greg and I were married following our move to the suburbs of Chicago, but all the love and security with which he provided me were not enough to soothe my nerves or calm my fears. Not only was I growing increasingly distraught over what Dr. Leonard had done to me, over the loss of my friends, and over the slowness with which the case was progressing, I was also being haunted by a lecture of Dr. Leonard's.

The words that rattled inside my brain had initially been spoken by Dr. Leonard as part and parcel of his lecture on Careers. Later, that portion of the lecture was segmented out from the rest and repeated to me as a casual reminder. Only now was I understanding the significance of his speech.

A man's career, he had said, was his chosen livelihood, and his livelihood was his means of survival. Without a livelihood, a man had no source of income, and without money, he could not survive in this society. Therefore, he reasoned out loud, anyone who attempts to interfere with the pursuit of another man's career is guilty of attempted murder, in that he threatens that man's existence. It followed, he went on, that if the threatened man kills the interfering source, it would not be murder, but self-defense.

There was no question that I had interfered with Dr. Leonard's career. And what I was recalling from my therapy now made me fear for my life. I had no doubts over whether Dr. Leonard *could* kill me; I had seen him beat a patient mercilessly, as well as display hand weapons on more than one occasion. I had no doubt that he *could* justify the act of killing me in his mind; he had already rationalized it in his lecture. I only questioned whether he *would*.

I told myself intermittently that I was being paranoiac. I told myself that no man in his right mind could really believe the syllogism that he had presented. But my fears subsided for only a flicker of time; I did not know if Dr. Leonard was in his right mind.

My fears worsened and my depression deepened, as I found myself capable of little else besides thoughts of the trial that was coming and the experiences that had passed. There were opportunities to put the anxiety of the upcoming trial behind me. Twice my lawyers had told me of rumblings from the other side to settle this case out of court. Neither time had I given it a moment's thought. I didn't want money. I wanted Dr. Leonard exposed. I rejected both offers. But keeping the issue alive in my mind and active in my life was not without its cost.

It became increasingly difficult for me to leave our apartment, as I was developing phobias about the environment that lay beyond my front door. I could not, for example, enter any high-rise structure or ride in an elevator without suffering an acute anxiety attack. I also developed an irrational fear of visible structures such as the suspensions that held bridges or the supports that ran through bleacher stands and sports stadiums. Driving over water or attending a football game became a major trauma for me. Tunnels that ran under rivers were often more intolerable than the bridges that spanned them, as I was certain that the structure that protected me would collapse and I would be drowned. Public places occupied by crowds filled me with terror, and the larger the crowd, the more overwhelming my anxiety. This resulted in my picking and choosing the hours for grocery shopping very carefully, as too many people in the market sent me home without any purchase.

Home was, during this time, the only place I wanted to be. It was the only place where I felt safe. There I could ponder the recent events of my life without interruption, hide from the rest of the world, and eat—which I did with increased frequency. Overeating had taken the place of near fasting and induced vomiting. And when errands did force me to venture out of the house, it was always with a pounding sense of urgency that I broke the speed limit to find my way home again, once my chore had been completed.

I knew that I needed help and that the suspicions I had grown to harbor about *all* psychiatrists and psychologists would have to be overcome. So I sought out the assistance of a clinic, where the expense of therapy would not be prohibitive and the environment of it would not be as threatening as a private practice. After being tested and interviewed at length, a procedure required before placement with a therapist could be made, the clinic informed me that my husband made just a bit too much money to qualify for treatment there. I did not understand why I had been made to wait a month and made to pay for the month's placement process, only to hear what could have been told to me upon filing my initial application. They referred me to an area psychologist in private practice and wished me well.

The psychologist agreed to accept insurance forms from Greg's company coverage in lieu of cash payments—the only way I could have undergone treatment at her price. After three sessions, she telephoned me at home to inform me that she had changed her mind and could not wait for payment to be processed through an insurance company. At such a desperate time of need, she discontinued my therapy and referred me back to the clinic.

This time, the clinic agreed to place me with a therapist, but informed me that that would take several weeks. It was not until months later, however, after Greg's work had taken us from Chicago to the South, that a letter was forwarded to our new home there: the clinic had a psychologist who was now ready to see me.

Greg remained patient and attentive during this entire period. He never pushed for a recovery that felt beyond my reach, or complained about the weight I was gaining. He always listened when I needed to talk, and always held me when I needed to cry. His love never wavered. Not once. If there was anything that carried me through those days that turned into years of waiting, it was him and the ever-present love and support he gave me. And it was the love I felt in return that made my survival of this bleak period seem worthwhile.

As the moment for Dr. Leonard's deposition grew closer, I wondered what explanation he would offer. I remembered having heard from some of his patients that he had exclaimed the psychological principles that had governed his behavior with me to be so complex that "they could fill an entire book." Then he implied his serious consideration of an attempt to do so. I tried to hypothesize now what great words might fill such a book, what great identifications he had made that had escaped so many others. I could fathom nothing save for what a madman or a simpleton might propose. So I returned to this puzzle again and again, in search of an answer I had perhaps overlooked.

I wondered what answers he could possibly give to the questions I hoped he would be asked at his deposition. I recalled the first night in his apartment and grew anxious to finally hear what the wrestling had meant and what his judgments on me had been. I recalled the night at the beach house and hoped that the questions he had dismissed then would be answered now. I remembered my summer employment in his apartment and the repeated instructions to swallow his semen in search of my own orgasm, and prayed that he would explain what *psychological principles* underlied those encounters. I recalled all the times I had questioned him, or tried to, in therapy sessions or in letters I wrote him, and hoped that my lawyers would get the answers I could not. I no longer needed just an understanding of past events, but an understanding of Dr. Leonard.

I did not entertain the possibility that he would deny the allegations against him. He had already implied acknowledgment of the accusations when he had told his questioning patients of the existence of a written consent form. I was certain that he would not risk the embarrassment of a reversal in strategy that might point to a contradiction in his words. It was for this same reason that I knew he would not allege insanity on my part as the cause for the legal action pending against him. That had been one of Patti's fears when she had contemplated suing him alone. It was never mine.

The Bill of Particulars alleged, among other things, that:

1. Negligence and malpractice took place from approximately January 1972 until approximately May 1977.

182

2. The negligent acts and/or omissions herein took place at the office, home, and summer house of the defendant.
3. The negligence, malpractice, and wrongdoing herein, consisted of: inducing the plaintiff to engage in various and sundry sexual relations with the defendant; in seducing the patient; in taking advantage of plaintiff's weakened psychological condition; in engaging in sexual intercourse with the plaintiff; in engaging in fellatio with the patient; in improper therapeutic, psychiatric, psychological and related therapy techniques; in deviating from customary and usual standards of practice; in failing to maintain proper professional detachment; in causing the plaintiff's psychological and/or psychiatric problems to be, become, and remain worse; and in failing to obtain a proper and informed consent.

It was now November 9, 1978, seven months since the dating of the Bill of Particulars, and Lonnie Franklin Leonard was present in the offices of Fuchsberg & Fuchsberg. This was the day he was to be questioned on all the allegations made against him. This was the day he would give explanations to all my remaining questions. This was the day of his deposition.

Mark Bower was the examining attorney for Fuchsberg & Fuchsberg. Acting as counsel for Dr. Leonard was Steven North of Garbarini, Scher & DeCicco. Present also was Dr. Leonard's third wife, the woman I had known as his girlfriend, Patricia Street.

It was quite early in the proceeding when the full extent of Dr. Leonard's confusion began to unravel. It was his testimony here that indicated that Nell and I had seen only the tip of the iceberg when we had discussed Dr. Leonard's confusion over the cosmetic bag and "the other woman" in his life.

(Mr. Bower is posing the questions. Dr. Leonard is giving the answers.)

Q Did you ever spend a night with this patient, regardless of who may have initiated such a—

A   Yes, I think that occurred once.
Q   When was that?
A   I have no idea.
Q   Did this happen at your office address or at some other location?
A   At some other location.
Q   Where was that?
A   It was in New Jersey.

Already I knew something was amiss. Why would he acknowledge one night, but not any of the others? If denial was going to be the basis of his defense, how could he hope that one exception would make any difference, especially when that one night was the first occasion of intercourse? The answers that Dr. Leonard continued to give began to explain this perplexity.

Q   Would you describe for me the circumstances by which you spent the night with the patient at this house?
A   As I recall, the patient called me at the end of my work week, on a Thursday evening, just when I was about to leave for a weekend at the Jersey Shore. She was complaining about feeling alone or depressed, or some other particular symptom that I can't specifically recall.
    I communicated to her that I was too tired to work anymore that week, could not. If she really needed medical attention, she would have to go to an emergency room or a hospital someplace in the neighborhood. That if she thought human companionship alone would be sufficient support she could accompany me there for the evening.
    She thought about it and made the choice to go along.
Q   Did you go with her to New Jersey?
A   Yes, if it doesn't make any difference whether I went with her or she went with me. She went with me.

184

Q Did you stay with her in the same house overnight?

A Yes.

Q Did you stay in the same bedroom overnight?

A I think at least part of the night might have been in the same bed. I don't recall.

Q Do you recall if she was dressed at that time?

A No, I don't.

Q Do you recall if you were dressed at that time?

A No, I don't.

Q Regardless of whether or not the two of you were dressed when you spent part of that night in the same bed, did you do that as part of your care and treatment of this patient?

A Already asked and answered. I was not working as a physician that night.

Q Was this entirely a social or personal matter in your perspective?

A Not in my perspective alone. It was explicitly defined to the patient that way.

Q During the course of that evening did you attempt to get the patient to have any physical contact with you?

A No.

Q Can you tell me how you spent the evening?

A Probably quietly watching TV or something. I don't recall.

At this point in Dr. Leonard's testimony, it did not occur to me that he was lying. Despite the contrary facts as I knew them, I could not conclude that Dr. Leonard was perjuring himself, because what he had just done was to describe a half true, incomplete story with which I was already very familiar: this was Linda's story! Dr. Leonard was, once again, confused and unable to recount, even in a procedure of this importance, what he had done to whom.

The line, however, between a confused mind and a blatant lie became less distinguishable as his testimony continued. Had he not been referring to my psychiatric file which he had carried with him, one might have been tempted to ask him several times during that day whether or not he was certain about which patient he was speaking.

> Q Did there come a time [when] you offered this patient employment?
> A Not that I recall.
> . . . Q Did you ever offer to employ her for housekeeping?
> A Not to my knowledge.

Did he really not remember? Could it be that he had forgotten an entire summer of my polishing pipes in the bathroom and fellating him in the bedroom? Or did he understand where an affirmative answer might lead in the questioning? It was still too early to determine if this was lunacy or blatant lying. I couldn't see any other choices.

What followed was questioning on the matter of informed consent. *Informed consent* in a case such as this would mean permission given either prior to or immediately following the commencement of therapy. It is the *informed* part of *informed consent* that requires it to be given so early in the psychotherapeutic process. Consent given at any later time risks the possibility, the probability, of the therapist influencing the patient's judgment and ultimate decision on the matter. The longer the patient has been in therapy, the longer her dependency on the therapist has had to develop, the greater the likelihood of such influence occurring. Under such circumstances, it is considered too high a probability that the patient will follow any course of treatment prescribed by her doctor, rather than the dictates of her pre-therapy values and better judgment. Permission extracted later in therapy is often obtained from a patient through psychological manipulation, and not as the result of an objective examination of the merits and risks of such "treatment."

But Dr. Leonard had received neither an early informed consent from me nor a later manipulated one. I had never signed any such statement. Now, however, he would finally explain what it was he had rationalized to his remaining patients to be my "written informed consent," or else acknowledge that no such consent had ever been given. He attempted the former, but accomplished neither.

> Q What I am asking is would it have been indicated to obtain a consent explicitly with respect to sexual contact?
> A It is a procedure that I would have taken.
> Q Did you ever obtain any explicit consent from [Ellen] to have sexual contact with you?
> A Yes.
> . . . Q Would you show me the consent form or the document which you maintain demonstrates her consent?
> A . . . It is an undated typewritten letter that I can only identify as an undated typewritten letter that in my files appears as one of the last communications from this patient.

The letter to which Dr. Leonard was referring was one in which I had expressed to him a desire to return to the time of protective embraces and parental hugs. In it I described to my therapist that those occasions of contact had made me feel "little, cozy, warm, and secure—very young." But the content of the letter was of far less significance than the timing of it.

> Q Did you receive any letters from her after you received this one?
> A No.
> Q Was this the last letter that you received from her?
> A Yes. As far as my records show.

The last letter written *before* this one *was* dated: December 3, 1976. An amateur sleuth could have placed the writing of the letter in question to be sometime after December 3, 1976, nearly five years *after* my therapy had begun, nearly four and a half years *after* fellatio had commenced, and nearly two years *after* intercourse had occurred! This was his document of informed consent! Dr. Leonard's continued testimony on this subject only served to underscore the absurdity of his position.

> Q Was she still your patient when you received this letter?
> A I don't know.

His pointing to a letter which was written at least two to four and a half years *after* the events for which the letter allegedly gave consent was irrational or stupid or both, I thought. But that I might not even have still been his patient, I thought made it insane.

Then the questioning turned to Dr. Leonard's *professional* opinions and diagnoses.

> Q Did you ever form an opinion or impression as to whether [Ellen] had formed any kind of dependency upon you arising from your professional relationship?
> A No, I formed no particular opinion about that.
> ... Q Did you ever form any opinion or impression as to whether, if you [were to have] sexual relations with this patient, it would be injurious to her mental health?
> A I don't recall forming any such an opinion.

But when that question was later posed in a slightly different form, Dr. Leonard changed his last answer.

> Q Did you ever form an opinion as to whether having sexual contact with this patient would be harmful to her mental condition?

A Yes. I formed the opinion that it would not.

He was also asked if, in his opinion, any acts he did with me were in my best interest. He answered that they were. Then he was asked:

> **Q** If you had any type of sexual contact with this patient, was that in the patient's best interest?
>
> **A** Yes.
>
> ... **Q** If it was your opinion that sexual therapy would have been of benefit to this patient, would it have been good practice for you to have followed that course of treatment?
>
> **A** Yes, and bad practice not to follow that—
>
> **MR. NORTH:** I move to strike that as gratuitous and not responsive.

But it wasn't until the questions put to Dr. Leonard focused on the sexual relationship between us that the true essence of his defense began to take form. With the first questions pertaining to fellatio, the mystery of what his book on psychological principles might contain began to unravel.

> **Q** Did there ever come a time that you—are you familiar with the term fellatio?
>
> **A** The term describing oral-genital sexual contact, yes.
>
> **Q** Did there ever come a time that you asked her to perform fellatio upon you?
>
> **A** No.
>
> **Q** Did there ever come a time that she, in fact, performed fellatio on you?
>
> **A** If you are using the term fellatio to describe a mutual pursuit of sexual pleasure, no. Whether there was oral-genital contact in the course of therapy, I am not certain.
>
> ... **Q** In what respect are you uncertain?

189

A I am not certain that it did occur.
Q Do you have any recollection if she ever took your penis into her mouth?
A No.

It took many more questions than the ones on fellatio, however, to paint the full picture of who this former giant among men truly was. It took over one hundred pages of testimony, splattered with questions about his sexual relationship with me, before his image began to shine through.

Q Were there ever any instances in which you took your clothes off in front of this patient?
A I don't recall.
. . . Q Did you ever lie on top of her?
A I don't recall.
. . . Q Did you ever penetrate her with your penis?
A I don't recall.
. . . Q Did she ever manually stimulate you sexually?
A I don't recall.

His answers to all such questions were consistent. They were summarized in one question and answer.

Q You have no specific recollection of any particular sexual acts [with] this patient; is that correct?
A That is correct.

Mr. Bower did not only question Dr. Leonard about encounters that had occurred, though, he also asked about events that had *not*. And for a purpose.

Q Doctor, did you ever perform cunnilingus on this patient?
A No.

. . . Q Can you explain to me how it is that you recall
that you never performed cunnilingus on this patient, but you do not recall that she performed fellatio on you?
MR. NORTH: Objection. That is his recollection.

With these answers, I was able to catch my first glimpse into
the mind of Dr. Leonard. I didn't get the answers to my questions concerning the unintelligible events of our relationship.
Perhaps that was what Tony had been trying to tell me when he
said that I would never understand them. Some behavior, some
events are not understandable by themselves. In order to make
sense of them, they must be considered in light of the irrational
source from which they come. When I could understand the
nature of the source, that it was irrational, I would stop looking
for sense in the actions themselves. That's what was happening
with the unfolding of Dr. Leonard's testimony. I was gaining an
insight into the man himself, and that would prove to be of
more benefit to me than I could imagine.

With all the time I had spent hypothesizing on what this day
would bring, what his explanations would be, what possible defense he might have chosen, I could never have foreseen the
answers that lie before me now. He could not recall if he had
been naked with me; he could not recall if he had lain on top of
me; he could not recall if he had been manually stimulated by
me; he could not recall if he had been fellated by me; he could
not recall if he had penetrated me—but *if* these things *had* occurred, he believed it would have constituted good therapy.
This was his line of defense. He had exceeded even my most
bizarre hypotheses.

Pretense at a failing memory was to be compounded by
more directly stated falsehoods before the questioning would
end. Any questions remaining on the character of the man
whom I had once believed to be so perfect, were resolved with
the end of his deposition.

Q Let us take the [last] time that she called [you]. Did she tell you why she was not coming back to you?
A No, she didn't.
Q Did you ask her?
A Yes.
Q What did she say in response to your inquiry?
A I don't recall exactly.
. . . Q Did she say anything about sexual contacts with you?
A I don't recall that.
Q Do you know why she left your care and treatment?
A No, I don't.

Again, I recalled the words he had spoken to me that morning over the phone: *I've suspected for a long time that what I have done to you has damaged you.* I remembered his insistence that I come to see him so that he might discuss in person my stated reasons for termination. I remembered, too, his replies of "I understand" to several of my explanations. The coffin on his honesty, on his integrity, had already been shut; he was simply hammering in the nails.

Q Did you ever spend a night with her other than the night in New Jersey?
A No.

How anxious I had been before this deposition to receive an explanation of his behavior during that first night in his apartment. But his denial that such a night, or any other night, ever occurred did not bar my understanding. It crystallized it. One of us, that night, had not been in control of our faculties, one of us had been unstable, one of us had been dangerous and destructive. And it wasn't the patient.

Q Did you ever achieve orgasm with her?
A No.

For a year and a half, I had given occasional thought to those patients of Dr. Leonard who had taken his side and condemned me in their letters and phone calls. I considered, on those occasions, what I might say to them, if I had had the opportunity: what logic I might employ to convince them of their error, what argument I might recite to expose Dr. Leonard's true nature. I would not spend any more time after today contemplating what scenarios I would write or what words I would say. Dr. Leonard had said it all.

15

FOUR ◇ YEARS
IN ◇ WAITING

The months passed slowly after Dr. Leonard's deposition. Occasionally, I occupied myself with the reading of his pre-trial examination. His words helped to ease the frustration of this long wait for trial, for at least I was waiting with new understanding. It was, for some reason, a strange consolation to hold that transcript in my hands and touch a bit of concrete evidence of a judgment made a year and a half ago. It did not lessen my impatience with this seemingly interminable procedure of civil justice; it simply eliminated the element of mystery that had previously surrounded his choice for a defense.

We were to remain in the Midwest for only another half year before Greg's work was to take us south, but those six months were marked by my first steps toward recovery—and more tragedy.

With Greg working nearly twelve hours a day and Eric, going on nine years old, occupied with school and extracurricular activities, it was time to find some productive outlet for myself. I wasn't ready for full-time employment in the real world of skyscrapers and crowds, so I started a small part-time business that could be run predominantly from my home.

It was my sister and my grandmother who provided an easy

move back into a limited social life. My sister and I had never been close as children, and when the final split had occurred between my parents and me, I fully anticipated that both she and my brother would follow the line of *loyalty to Mother*, which we had all been taught, but which I alone had been unable to swallow. Whereas my brother stood steadfast by that lesson, my sister sought me out some months after the split, and our relationship seemed to be making up for lost time ever since.

Her ties to home, however, were never broken. At best, they were slightly stretched when she finally moved out on her own in her late twenties. She moved only as far as across the street from her parents, but at least she moved. With her strings tied so tight to a place I saw as so destructive, I questioned how far our own friendship might develop. But the questions never kept me from pressing for as much closeness as I could get now. And I think, for the first time in our lives, we grew to love each other.

Grandma, however, was the true force behind my selection of the Chicago suburbs for my home after New York. It was not that she advocated the relocation. It was merely her presence that brought me back. Besides needing to be in a place that was familiar, I needed to be where I knew I was loved—loved in a parental, protective kind of way. That was with my grandma. The timing of my choice for both of us could not have been better.

Whereas I never told Grandma of the treatment I had received from Dr. Leonard, or of my lawsuit against him now, we still shared more during those months than we had ever shared before. I seized the opportunity of my return to visit with her often and to bring her pleasures for which others seemed too busy. Often that would include driving her downtown for an afternoon of shopping and a long lunch, or picking her up only to drive back out to the suburbs for dinner at her favorite restaurant. She never knew how difficult these excursions away from home were for me, but she appreciated them as if she did.

Whatever the occasion of our visit was, we talked seriously and in depth, as if we both knew that each time might be our last. It was during some of these visits that our conversations about my mother and father became more explicit, more honest, than they had been during my adolescence. She told me that she always felt an undercurrent of hatred from my mother toward her, and that underneath her facade of smiles and small talk, my mother detested every moment she ever spent in Grandma's presence.

"It's not the hatred I mind so much," she explained to me. "It's that she won't say what I did that made her hate me so. Maybe if she told me, we could talk about it."

"That's never been her way, Grandma. It's always been easier for her to pretend one thing, while delivering a contradictory message in more subtle ways," I offered in support of her suspicions.

She told me how difficult that had been for her to handle. She had often wondered if she wasn't reading something into my mother's behavior that really wasn't there. "Tell me," she asked me once, "were my feelings right, or was I crazy?"

My God, I wondered, how many years has my mother had my grandmother doubting *her* sanity? "You weren't crazy, Grandma," was all I said. I did not tell Grandma just how often my mother had expressed contempt for her in the privacy of our own apartment, or how often I listened to the words of dread as Mommy prepared for a visit to Grandma's home. But what I did say was enough to confirm her feelings, validate her emotional sensitivity, and help her to relieve any lingering doubts about herself.

It was mostly during my visits to her apartment that I became privy to the secrets of her life, the intimacies of her marriages, and the sorrows of her two exposures to widowhood. She shared with me, too, the disappointments and frustrations of her third and present marriage, in a way that made me cry for this woman's loneliness. And in the most solemn of our moments together, she would reach across the sofa where we were both seated and take my hand in hers, and cry quietly as she expressed her deepest fears about dying. These, perhaps, were the moments I cherished most, not only because she could share her pain, but because she was so open and vulnerable with me—and, too, because these were the moments when I was freest to show her how much I loved her.

"Grandma," I whispered to her once while she cried, "I would love to return to a time when we were both younger. I would tell you that you will never die, and I would say so because I would not want to believe otherwise. But if I told you that now, you would never trust me enough to cry with me in the future. Instead, all I can tell you is that, even if your life ended tomorrow, the love I have always felt for you would live inside me forever. I don't know if that makes it easier for you. I don't know if there's anything I could say that would. I can only tell you that it is the truth."

The look she returned in answer to my statement told me that, indeed, I had eased some of her pain. At least, temporarily. We had several moments like this one before she died in January of 1979, and after her passing, I never had one moment's regret over things not said or feelings not spoken. There was, unfortunately, one instance of regret over something not done.

I was standing over Grandma's bed in the intensive care ward, holding her hand in frustrated awareness that there was nothing I could do to help her in her final day. She was bitterly aware of everything going on: the pipe that had been placed down her throat that prevented her from speaking, the tubes that kept her from moving freely, and the indignity of not being able to void in the privacy of a bathroom. She signaled for a paper and pen, then wrote me a note asking for another pillow. One was brought.

But when my mother walked into the room, moved to the side of the bed where I was standing, looked down into Grandma's eyes and smiled that syrupy smile of sympathy and concern, I was paralyzed.

"She knows you don't mean it!" I cried in my mind. But I couldn't get the words out. "This is no time for fakery!" I thought. I wanted to make these the first words I would have spoken to my mother in three years, but my voice remained silent.

Truth and honesty were not even sacred at death. It felt blasphemous! The ultimate insult! And I was incapable of doing anything about it.

I looked at my grandmother, and she at me, while my mother's transparent smile never broke. Grandma's eyes looked yearning and pained. They told me how much she wanted to be able to speak. I interpreted her look to say, "Why won't you do something to stop this charade?" But that was not my grandmother's eyes talking, that was my guilt. I'd like to think that what she really wanted to tell me was, "It's okay." But I'll never know for sure. She died the next morning.

We had just relocated to Tampa, Florida, when I was called to give my deposition in July of 1979. In the very room in which Dr. Leonard had been examined, I was questioned by the same attorney who had, in the previous session, acted as Dr. Leonard's counsel. And, with all the gentleness, grace, and delicacy of a bull in a china shop, Steven North questioned me for nearly seven hours not only about my five and a half years with Dr. Leonard, but about my childhood, my employment history, and my sex life, as well. He did so in a tone that accused, badgered, or snickered. Besides listening to and answering his inquiries in these sensitive areas of my past and present, I also had to listen, without any visible response, to his offhanded sarcastic remarks.

(Mr. Douglas is acting as counsel for the plaintiff. Mr. North is posing the questions and acting on behalf of the defendant.)

Q   You then [lay] down on the couch?
A   There was no couch.

MR. DOUGLAS: *[Lay]* down on the couch.

MR. NORTH: I guess in this case, yes.
MR. DOUGLAS: No. That's proper grammar.

But there were several questions that I found most revealing. They told me of the defense's concern over Dr. Leonard's words to me during our last telephone conversation: *I've suspected for a long time that what I have done to you has damaged you.* The questions did not come together, but were separated by questions relating to other matters. And two of those questions were, I thought, more obvious than the others.

> Q   At the time you spoke to Dr. Leonard, after you last saw him in or about May of 1977, was anyone else party to that telephone conversation, either by listening or by speaking, other than you and Dr. Leonard?

And the very last question I was asked that day, I believe, expressed concern over those same words.

> Q   Did you ever tape a conversation with Dr. Leonard?

Unfortunately, I had not.

I returned to Tampa that evening feeling as if I'd been beaten up, but having no visible bruises to show for my ordeal. I collapsed in my son's bedroom, which was vacant for the summer while he visited with his father in Connecticut, and cried alone for the entire night. Greg tried to comfort me, but this was a time that could not be shared with any other human being. I had been alone in what Dr. Leonard had done to me, and I was alone now in what I had chosen to do about it.

In seven hours, I had relived the five and a half years I had spent with Dr. Leonard; in seven hours, I had exhumed the details of my childhood; in seven hours, I had told a hostile stranger intimate details of my sex life. During those seven hours, I listened to questions that contained twisted facts or half-truths, ignored context, and insinuated accusations of immoral, and even criminal conduct, just by the way the questions were phrased. I had already been instructed by my attorney to answer only the question that was put to me, and to volunteer no more than the question required. So I had to swallow my impulse to make corrections and object to innuendos.

Now every fiber of my being was feeling what I could not allow myself to feel during those seven hours: the pain of my relationship with Dr. Leonard, the pain of my childhood and more recent family rejections, the pain of sharing intimacies I regarded as private—and the pain of being treated, once again, as if it was *I* who had done something wrong. No words could have conveyed what those seven hours had been like, nor my fear at going through it again at trial. Only I could experience and appreciate how far down all this went, and know that, in this absolute worst of all my moments, it would have to be endured alone.

In the year that followed my deposition, I tried once again to put the matter of Dr. Leonard and the pending trial behind me. With great trepidation over facing the more real world, I registered for the spring term at the state university as a second-semester sophomore. Greg drove me to the school several times, so that I would not fear the drive to an unknown place, and so that I could ease into the adjustment of being with larger groups of people. Together, we mapped out the location of the buildings in which my classes would be conducted, and made the trip to each building so that I would feel confident of making the trip alone. When the time came for classes to commence, I vowed to put everything else on a back burner in my mind, and I plunged into my school work with eagerness and excitement.

I continued to think about the lawsuit almost daily, but it did not consume me nor preoccupy my thoughts, as it had in the past. Only at New Year's Eve did I feel the frustration of how long the suit had dragged on, as each year I phoned my lawyers at this time to ascertain the status of the case. Each time, I was told that the trial would "probably be sometime this year." And each year's ending would tell me that they had been wrong. Were it not for the goals I saw being served by the trial, I might have considered abandoning the suit just to have the whole matter over and done with. But I was motivated to keep going by the knowledge that desertion of my goals would leave me unsettled for a much longer time than that for which I had waited for trial. The goals were few and simple. The first was to exercise some control in a relationship previously dictated by Dr. Leonard. To maintain the silence he had exacted from me for so many years meant that he still controlled me. To speak out in naming what he did and what he was, had less to do with the consequences that I hoped would befall Dr. Leonard than it had to do with reasserting the strength of my spirit, which I needed to believe had not been irreparably crippled.

I also needed to have the facts of what had occurred between us transcribed into a permanent form. The only honest record of what had occurred for five and a half years was carried within me. I could not risk that coming years and fading memories might invalidate the pain I had experienced and the cruelty he had perpetrated. I wanted to take the information I carried and put it in a place outside of myself. I wanted to say the words aloud and know that they were heard. I wanted to testify.

The decision to resume my education had been the right one. The pressures of academic achievement not only shifted my focus away from the pending trial and past tribulations, it afforded me the opportunity to demonstrate my long-dormant abilities, and to test my determination to recover from the dependency and depression that had become my way of life. By the time I graduated less than two years later, I had a record of high academic achievement behind me, acceptances into graduate schools, the satisfaction of new friendships, a renewed self-confidence, and an absolute certainty that I was now capable of determining my own destiny. It was not that all my fears had been eliminated. They hadn't. It was that they were no longer running my life.

*   *   *

Anne Kaplan was Associate and Trial Associate with Fuchsberg
& Fuchsberg. It was she whom I called before New Year's each
December, and it was she who always reassured me when I
grew tired of waiting. Now, only three months after my gradua-
tion, she was calling to inform me of the last step in the series of
procedures before trial. On March 26, 1982, the Medical Malpractice Mediation Panel would convene to hear both sides in
all the cases against Lonnie Franklin Leonard, M.D. The function of this panel, consisting of a judge, a lawyer, and a physician, would be to make a determination of *Liability* or *No
Liability* in the case of this defendant.

For a finding of liability, the panel would have to affirma-
tively decide two factors: (1) that the treatment rendered by the
doctor was a departure from good medical practice, and (2) that
the treatment was the cause of injury to the patient. An affirmative determination on one factor alone would be insufficient
to render the physician liable.

In cases where the physician denies the treatment of which
he is accused, the panel is unable to determine liability. In fact,
the panel is obliged to refuse a decision in the matter. Only if
the doctor acknowledges the treatment of which he is accused,
and either defends it or refutes the allegation that it was the
cause of injury to the patient, can the panel hear and judge the
case.

If the panel *unanimously* decided liability in our cases
against Dr. Leonard, the finding could be entered as evidence at
the trial. Anne Kaplan explained that such evidence would
carry the same weight as testimony from an expert witness. It
was clearly a decision for which we all hoped. And with one
exception, none of us were disappointed. In all but Patricia Osborne's case, the panel had unanimously judged liability in the
cases against Dr. Leonard.

Patti's case now stood unique among the rest of ours. It was
not that the panel had ruled differently in her case, it was that
they were unable to rule at all. In this one case, Dr. Leonard

202

denied the "treatment" of which he was accused, barring the panel's judgment. We all attributed his denials in Patti's case to one more example of his confusion over what he had done to whom. In all the other cases, however, he had acknowledged the specified "treatment" and had unsuccessfully tried to defend it, or argue that it was not the cause of the resulting injuries. Because the panel hearings and records are closed, we were unable to ascertain the exact nature of his position.

Besides the panel finding Dr. Leonard liable in all the cases on which it could rule, the outcome also determined the order in which the cases would be tried. Since "treatment" was being denied by Dr. Leonard in Patti's case, hers would go first.

During all my telephone conversations with Anne Kaplan over the years, she had often answered my impatience with the plodding court system, by reminding me that once a firm trial date was set and kept, the speed with which the cases would proceed would be lightning fast. But after five years of waiting, and after four more months of postponed trial dates, I found it hard to believe, when Anne called me on October 29, 1982, to beckon me to New York, that this was really it. The jury, she offered in proof, had been selected that day.

"Plan to stay for a couple of weeks," she advised. First, I would serve as a witness in Patti's case, she said, and then as the plaintiff in my own.

This was when I first learned that there were only three suits still outstanding against Dr. Leonard. One of the five had been dropped when the dates of Dr. Leonard's treatment of the plaintiff were found to have passed the Statute of Limitations. And Linda, Anne told me, had dropped her case against Dr. Leonard at the eleventh hour, just prior to the commencement of trial, and without any explanation. It was assumed by us all that her earlier fear of publicity had won out.

As I packed my suitcase and the imminence of the trial became real to me, I was filled with apprehension and fear: apprehension over a repeat of the publicity these cases had received in 1977, and fear over the prospect of reliving my deposition on the witness stand. Then I thought about facing Dr. Leonard. I thought about his lecture on Careers and wondered if he would try to hurt me. I thought about his bug eyes and wondered if he would still be able to intimidate me after all these years just by staring at me. I thought about his power over me in the past and wondered if seeing him again would resurrect any reflex of obedience to him. And with these thoughts, I understood for the first time the terror that fills a rape victim at confronting her assailant. It was more than the fear of him and what he could do to me; it was the fear of what I might be capable of in order to prevent him from doing it again.

I assured myself that my fears were founded merely on the illusion of his power which he had taught me, and on the intensity of my contained rage—not on any real threats that existed. He could not hurt me there, and I knew I could not be provoked to violence. By the time I boarded the plane on Monday, my fear had been replaced with an undercurrent of calm: an end to these eleven years was now in sight.

16

OSBORNE VS. LEONARD

Tuesday morning, the day before court reconvened, I met the Partner and Trial Counsel with Fuchsberg & Fuchsberg, Edwin N. Weidman. It was he who would handle our cases in court. Together, we reviewed Dr. Leonard's psychiatric record on me, a file I was seeing for the first time. As Ed Weidman examined this record for possible areas of cross-examination, I looked with incredulity at the pages of notes and at what Dr. Leonard had chosen to include or exclude from these entries on my progress. Under the date stamped April 5, 1972, he had written: *bedded down for the nite* (sic). He did not, however, identify what he had done to me that first night in his apartment, nor was there any mention of the beach house session, nor was there a record of the location of the December 1976 sessions which had occurred in my bedroom. When the notes had been thoroughly reviewed and the missing information filled in for Ed, I felt ready to face the defense lawyer, the jury, and even Dr. Leonard.

A quiet discussion at the bench began the day's work in court on Wednesday morning. Dr. Leonard was nowhere to be seen, and that was the topic of discussion between the lawyers and the judge.

(George J. Kehayas, of Garbarini, Scher & DeCicci, is acting as Trial Counsel for the defense.)
MR. KEHAYAS: . . . Dr. Leonard informed me that he was
returning to his home in Florida, he did not intend to testify
in this case nor in any other cases, that he saw no purpose in
continuing his preparation for testimony in this case . . .

When this inaudible discussion had terminated, and the
judge called for the jury's return to the courtroom, Ed informed
us of Dr. Leonard's decision, and then excused me from the
courtroom. I would not, he explained, be privy to the trial's
disclosures until after I had testified. For the time being, I was
to wait outside in the corridor while Patti took the stand.
It had been the Friday before when Ed Weidman had introduced Patti's case to the jury. During his opening statement, he
explained to the jury, among other things, the phenomenon of
transference and how it related to the matter at hand.

. . . Now, the important ingredient in this phenomenon of
transference is that it's recognized as what happens to [the
patient], but it's the physician who must maintain detachment.
. . . [H]e must never permit social contact with his patient[s] . . . because they are seeking help, because they are
making [him] into a demigod, because they do believe [what
the therapist says] is for their best interest and they will act
upon what [he is] suggesting or what [he is] directing.
. . . Whether [sexual contact with the therapist] is during [a]
therapy session, before a therapy session, or after a therapy
session, it's unethical, it's improper, it's wrong, and it's
damaging.
Now, that sort of conduct . . . can take the form of as-
sault, it can take the form of seduction, it can take the form
of manipulation of the patient's conduct. And that is what
we are concerned with.

Now Patti was inside the courtroom detailing her experiences with Dr. Leonard.

(Ed Weidman is posing the questions. Patti is providing the answers.)

Q And on how many days or occasions that you can recall [did you have] oral sex with him?
A It was weekly, over a couple of months.
Q And when did this come about: before, during, or after each of the sessions?
A After.

Soon the questioning turned to the derepression sessions.

Q Tell us, when you had these [derepression] sessions, where were you and what did you do?
A To make me feel the most helpless, and I guess uncomfortable, [I would] be on the floor of his office naked and spread-eagle.
Q And for how long were you in that position, naked and spread-eagle, during these sessions?
A For the fifty-five minutes.
Q And where was the doctor during these sessions?
A Sitting next to me.
Q And how was he dressed?
A He was naked.

Then Mr. Weidman directed Patti from a general discussion of derepression sessions to one in particular which had been critical for her.

Q Now, let's come to this time, I think you say in March of 1974. It's a primal therapy session?
A Yes.
Q Okay. Tell us what happened on that day.

A It's very difficult to lie spread-eagle and naked. And at that point in time I was—I just couldn't do it, so I just knelt down, withdrew into—a fetal position with my head down, and out of the clear blue sky, Dr. Leonard, entered me from behind. He put his penis in my vagina.

Q And when he did that, did he ejaculate into your vagina?

A Yes.

Q Did he say anything to you before this happened?

A No.

Q Did he say anything to you after this happened?

A No, sir.

While Patti continued with her testimony, I waited outside the courtroom, occasionally looking through the glass window on the courtroom door to see how Patti was holding up, or down the corridor for signs of Dr. Leonard, who I still believed was going to appear. I waited like this all day, and when Ed Weidman and Patti emerged from the courtroom at the end of the day, she still had not finished. She would take the stand again the next morning.

On Thursday morning, I waited again in the corridor for Patti to finish. This day, however, I did not wait alone. Nell and Marta, former patients of Dr. Leonard who had agreed to testify, kept me company. Nell's testimony was important because her Ph.D. in mathematics and conservative demeanor made the point that neither extraordinary intelligence nor a discriminating attitude protected female patients from Dr. Leonard. Marta's testimony, however, served another purpose. Her testimony presented a new dimension of Dr. Leonard's character. Nell testified after Patti, with Marta following only twenty minutes later. I was to testify last.

(Mr. Weidman is posing the questions. Marta is providing the answers.)

Q   And when you came to see Dr. Leonard, did he take you in as a patient?

A   Yes, he did.

Q   And was there a time that you had, or there was rather, sexual contact between you and the doctor?

A   Yes, there was.

Q   Would you tell us when, where and how, please?

A   Should I give the full story of what happened?

Q   Yes, please.

A   Tell everything?

Q   Yes.

A   Okay.

THE COURT: When was it? Let's start with that.

A   In the fall of 1974. He had invited my mother and my-self down to his beach house for the weekend at Point Pleasant, New Jersey, along with Pat Street.

Friday night he offered to drive me down to the beach house; my mother could not make it until the following day. Neither could Pat. No one was at the house. So, we drove down Friday night.

Saturday morning when I awakened—the bedrooms were—there was a wall adjoining the bedrooms and from his room he asked me if I wanted to come and get in bed with him when we first woke up in the morning. And I said, "No. No, I don't really want that. No thank you. I am fine here."

Later that morning, I put my bathing suit on to go to the beach and to walk on the beach, beyond the beach, go into the water. And he had on his jogging shorts like a bathing suit. And when I came back into the house, he took me into the bedroom that I had been staying in and told me that he was going to show me the difference in the feelings that I was experienc-ing in my life. The difference of feelings between being a little girl and the difference between being a grown woman.

At first he started to tickle me, and this was on the bed. He asked me to lie down on the bed. I was on the bed and he started to tickle me, and I started to giggle. And he said, "This is what it's like to be a little girl." And he stopped after a while.

And then he started to rub his hands all over my body. And several times he got his whole body on top of mine and started massaging me and rubbing me all over and saying, "This is what it's like to feel like a woman." And then he would stop.

And then he started tickling me again and I started laughing. And he said, "This is what it's like to be a little girl." And he would stop.

And then he would get on top of me, or he would rub me again, and he would say, "This is what it's like to be a woman."

And this went on for over an hour. A while over an hour. I would say two hours.

It was not *this* content of Marta's testimony that had the most impact. Dr. Leonard had done far worse to others. What made the disclosures of Dr. Leonard's actions so astounding in this case, was Marta's age when the incident occurred. She had been fourteen years old!

The conclusion of Marta's testimony seemed as good a time as any to break. Court was recessed till two o'clock. I would testify after lunch.

After the others had taken their seats inside, Ed Weidman emerged from the courtroom.

"The defense made an offer to settle Patti's case during lunch," he told me. "Mr. Kehayas cannot, however, settle Patti's case without yours." Here we were, in the middle of trial, just moments away from my testifying, and the lawyers were talking settlement. I could not understand this.

"I thought cases were supposed to be settled *before* trial, not during trial," I said.

"It doesn't always happen that way," he explained.

"But I told you in the beginning, Ed, that I didn't want to settle. I just want Dr. Leonard to be exposed and I want to be heard."

Anne Kaplan arrived at the courthouse just in time to witness this development. Anne had always understood my feelings about this case. She had been able to address herself logically to what I had been too emotional to comprehend without her assistance. It was she to whom I turned now for guidance.

"You have been heard, Ellen," she told me. "First of all, your deposition is public record. More than that, though, is that none of these other women would be here today if it hadn't been for you. Their testimony and yours have exposed Dr. Leonard. And you made that happen."

"But I want more, Anne," I told her. "I want to testify in front of a jury—a group of normal people, not Objectivists— and have them say out loud that what Dr. Leonard did was wrong."

"If the jury found for you and against Dr. Leonard, would that really tell you anything you already didn't know?" she asked. It was not unusual, she told me, for a plaintiff to desire much more from a lawsuit than what a civil suit was designed to provide. An action such as this one, she went on to say, will not result in giving back the years Dr. Leonard took away. It will not remove the pain he inflicted or the damage he has done. It won't even punish him for what he did: he will not go to jail and he will not even pay the damages out of his own pocket. Nor will he even lose his license to practice medicine or psychotherapy in the future. Even if Patti's case went full course, and mine followed after hers, this kind of satisfaction would never be mine. All that a malpractice suit can do, she explained, is award some amount of financial compensation for the suffering and injury sustained by the plaintiff.

"But I want to testify, Anne," I pleaded. "I've waited five and a half years just to say in court what he's done to me, what kind of man he is."

She understood. So did Ed. They offered to let me testify even if the case was settled, promising to withhold the case's resolution from the jury.

"But it won't mean anything to the outcome of the case if it's been resolved."

Anne and Ed urged me not to let this factor affect my decision. If I wanted to testify, I could, but a rational decision about settlement should not take into account any other issue than what amount of money, in the context of precedents and reasonable expectations, would *feel* closest to a satisfactory compensation.

"What did they offer Patti?" I asked Ed in defeat. I knew already from the way he was talking to me that whatever the amount was, he thought it was a fair settlement.

"One hundred thousand dollars," he answered.

"And what did they offer me?"

"They want to know what it will take, but I'm certain they're prepared to pay the same thing to you," he replied. "And that really is a fair amount, Ellen."

I thought about what he and Anne had said. For the first time, I saw that this day for which I had waited so long, concerned itself with little else than dollars and cents. How much more noble the system had seemed when I believed it might establish proper standards of conduct for physicians and protection for female patients and a forum for the exposure of evil therapists. But Anne had been wrong; money would not be the only thing I would have to show for this lawsuit. Dr. Leonard's practice was closed; he had been named for what he was; he no longer benefited from the unquestioning loyalty and adoration of so many people, which had come his way for so many years. And I—I had reaffirmed my spirit. I had been strong enough to fight my therapist and determined enough to see it through to the end. The Dr. Leonards of the world didn't even show up for battle. He had closed up shop, run off to Florida, and still had not made an appearance at the trial against him.

"One hundred and fifty thousand dollars," I said to Ed, "and

I'll think about testifying in the event they agree to that amount." I knew they would never agree. I knew I would still testify, and it would not be to a mock court.

"One hundred and fifty thousand?" he exclaimed. "Ellen, be reasonable."

I'm being as reasonable as Dr. Leonard's treatment of me was, I thought. "That's the minimum I can accept, Ed," I told him resolutely.

Ed reappeared almost as quickly as he had left. He was smiling as he extended both his hands in signal to extend mine to him. When my hands were tightly gripped in his, he looked right at me and said simply, "It's all over."

I thought I understood the meaning of what he was saying, but I was not sure. "You mean they said 'yes'?"

"They said 'yes.'"

I began to sob. In the most spontaneous and intense flow of emotion I had ever experienced, I began to sob uncontrollably. I had never given any thought to what the end would feel like. I guess I never believed there would be an end. Now, in this final moment, there was no room for thought, only feeling. I hadn't known how much tension had resulted from the last five and a half years until, through my tears, it found its release. And I hadn't known that without testifying, I could feel what I was feeling now: victorious.

I had not stopped crying when I became aware of a conspicuous absence. The women with whom I should have been sharing this time were nowhere to be seen.

"Where are the witnesses? Where's Patti?" I was asking Ed through my tears. Why weren't they here, I wondered.

"They're still in the courtroom, but first you'd better calm—"

I never heard the second half of his message. I was running into the courtroom. When I had spotted the back of Marta's blond head, I cried out to her, "It's over, Marta! It's finally over."

Marta, Nell, and Patti ran to where I was standing, and as

they hugged me and one another, they, too, began to cry. And in this rush of tears, hugs, and laughter, I had not noticed the judge, the jury, and the defense counselor were all in their appropriate places, as if expecting to proceed. I did not know it, but all except Mr. Kehayas were unaware of what had transpired. Even Patti had not yet been told. It was not until I heard the sound of the gavel several minutes after our celebration had begun, that I looked up to discover their presence, and to discover all eyes upon us—many of which were filled with tears.

"That's what I was trying to tell you," I heard Ed say from behind me as he placed his hand on my shoulder.

This time, when court was called to order, I asked Ed for permission to leave. I found my way to a telephone booth at the end of the hall.

"Greg?" I was still crying. "It's all over. It's finally over. And I'm coming home."

"Use some of that money to get some therapy," a man's voice was saying from behind me. "After what was done to you, you'll need help in straightening it all out." The psychiatrist whom Ed Weidman had intended to call as our expert witness was offering what he believed was good advice as we were leaving the courthouse. His suggestion made me want to laugh and punch his face, all at the same time. Therapy? Psychotherapy? Never. Never again, I thought. I never want to see another therapist as long as I live!

The trial was over, but somehow things did not yet feel totally complete. The psychiatrist's suggestion had bothered me, but not nearly as much as my strong and sweeping internal response to it. I knew I still had unfinished business. And by the time I boarded my return flight to Tampa, I knew what the business was. I needed an understanding of how it had all happened. Was it all a product of Dr. Leonard's own brand of evil? Or, perhaps, was it sickness? How much of a role had Objectivism played in making this all possible? And how much was attributable to *real* problems I had that made me prey to the likes of a Dr. Leonard? I knew that all these questions would need answers if I was to ever feel confident that nothing like this could ever happen to me again. Not having the answers made me feel uncomfortably vulnerable and stood in the way of a true sense of finality.

I knew that without Dr. Leonard, the unique nightmare that was mine would not have come to pass. Had my therapist been competent, professional, moral, and sane, no other contributing factors alone would have borne such ill results. Whether his was a case of lunacy or evil, I never figured out. It stopped seeming important after a while. The answer would not have altered the outcome.

The roles of Objectivism and Objectivists seemed inseparable as I contemplated their separate effects on past events. Ayn Rand had carefully guarded the term *Objectivist*, reserving it only for those deserving few who she felt had earned it. But Dr. Blumenthal had been appointed such a worthy party, and his behavior with me had been so contemptible that Mr. Fuchsberg had considered making him a co-defendant in the malpractice suit. Only for fear of diluting the bigger issue had the idea been dropped.

My friends and acquaintances, the students of Objectivism, behaved no more honorably, independently, bravely, than did the Objectivist, Dr. Blumenthal. They spoke eloquently about morality, ethics, and independent thinking. But being loyal to Objectivism and to their Objectivist psychiatrist kept them from practicing at least the last, just as it had me for so long. Further, being so loyal seemed to convince them that they were all the more ethical, moral, and independent for being so. I had once known that delusion as well.

The numbers of these blindly devoted went beyond coincidence. There was more to this than just a chance meeting of several dozen sheep all willing to follow their *hero*, their *ideal man* anywhere. Maybe the "hook" was in the lesson that if Objectivism was the right way, then being a student of Objectivism made us more right than others. And for those of us who were not certain of our value to begin with, such superiority helped us to ignore our self-evaluations and feed our egos.

But maybe it was in Ayn Rand's separation of *Objectivists* who were fit to provide the answers, from the *students of Objectivism* who were qualified only to ask—and the acceptance by both groups of their proper assigned function. Such segregation of those who knew from those who didn't, certainly led the way for Dr. Leonard to assume the same authority without expectation of rebellion from his patients.

Or maybe it was in Ayn Rand's incorporation of "hero-worship" into her representation of romantic love; show an Objectivist a hero and the hero has but to take or command. In Ayn Rand's novel *The Fountainhead*, the heroine is raped by the book's hero, "(b)ut," Ms. Rand wrote in the scene, "the act of a master taking shameful contemptuous possession of her was the kind of rapture she had wanted." How many of Dr. Leonard's victims had known such rapture? How many had been taught, either through Ms. Rand's words or Dr. Leonard's actions, that in such an act, they should? How many had tried to believe and come to accept that *this* was the standard by which to evaluate femininity and mental health? That this was the goal for which to strive in their therapy?

I didn't know all the answers then. I still don't. But I felt there was something in the philosophy itself that both attracted people like Dr. Leonard, and blinded a group of otherwise highly intelligent, well-motivated people. Somewhere in her writing, Ayn Rand had unwittingly laid the foundation for a cult.

Added to the philosophy was a dimension given by the students themselves: the creation of a hero beyond judgment. At risk of losing all of one's friends and acquaintances, one could make a negative judgment of Dr. Leonard. So it was, too, for negative judgments on a designated Objectivist. Any of their flaws that were too blatant to be ignored were always to be weighed against the benefit of their contributions. (Is that not what Dr. Leonard had counted on the evening following his Christmas party?) What did that say about the contributions of the rest of us? The bottom line was: one group was perfect or excusably tarnished; the other group was still proving the value of their presence on this earth.

Objectivism played into both sides of the self-doubt coin. It told us we were better than others for we had found the truth, but it kept us in constant fear of being judged as less good than what we should be, the consequence of which was abandonment. And it reminded us with labels like "student" and "patient" that we had not yet arrived. If, however, we worked hard enough, if we were moral enough, if we were good enough, someday someone else would let us know we had. Dr. Leonard capitalized on it all.

But Objectivism and therapy had not occurred in a vacuum. I brought to them a breeding ground for exploitation that had been my upbringing. And in this sense, my experience with Dr. Leonard was unique. I supposed that a good case could be made for the similarity between the way that Dr. Leonard had led me to view his sexual escapades with me and the way that my father had explained his treatment of me that night in the maid's room. Each man tried to teach me that just by virtue of his saying so and his position of authority, he had done nothing wrong; and that by virtue of my upset over their treatment of me, I had. My father labeled my perceptions and memories inaccurate; Dr. Leonard labeled my reactions and emotions neurotic. And each was totally convinced that he had placed blame for any problems between us on the right place: my mind.

Each also taught me in his own way that his actions toward me set me apart from others and made me "special" in his eyes.

Even more similar, however, were the daily contradictions between how each of these men acted and the words of reason and logic they professed to believe. While both men were stu-

217

dents of the same philosophy, my father personified the loyal servant, while Dr. Leonard reigned as master over his faithful following, neither an example of what they preached. *Any* person would have been confused, much less one who was being taught to doubt her own feelings and thinking processes.

Dr. Leonard's similarity to my mother was, in hindsight, just as striking. How brilliantly each sought to control me, each by professing to know my inner thoughts and feelings better than I, each teaching me to doubt my perceptions and processes. Dr. Leonard was able to succeed where my mother had failed *only* because I trusted him. With my mother, I always knew better.

But I don't believe it was the similarity between parents and therapist that alone set the groundwork for such abuse from Dr. Leonard. Transference helped, but it did not suffice. It could not, by itself, explain my groveling in my probation session, or my hoping to earn *my* way back into *his* good graces. What was needed was a fundamental belief in the lessons that were taught to the child I had been, which I was so certain had been discarded along the way. Intellectually, they had been. But in a place inside me so deep that its existence had been unknown, I had believed every word of my mother's lessons: I was not sane, I was not good, and I was not worthy of being loved. Dr. Leonard had only to nod at any one of these, and I, trusting him so, was reduced to the helplessness I had felt as the child first learning these lessons from my mother.

Then there were the lessons I learned from my father. Approval came from letting yourself be used, and remaining loyal to the user. It came from being an independent thinker, yet following all the rules of an insane household. And approval came from being willing to let the offender pretend that the offense was something else. My father had taught me all of that. And love—love came from following orders. With my mother's help, my father had taught me that, too.

Dr. Leonard, a philosophy turned into a cult, and an upbringing that could not have better set the stage for the events in my twenties had it been deliberately designed that way, all played a role in the drama that consumed my life for so many years. The trial ended only the drama. It took many more months of answering these questions to feel complete and finished with it all.

For my own part, there were two lessons learned well. Never, never again would I let anyone tell me they know me better than I know myself. I have learned to trust my emotions—and to act on them. The slightest twinge from my gut that tells me the person I am dealing with is not honest, good, and stable, puts my guard up or sends me running in the opposite direction. Eventually, I'm usually proven right.

And I have learned to never tolerate abuse that goes unapologized for or unacknowledged. Not sexual, physical, nor verbal abuse. Those who expect such leeway in life may feel themselves privileged and above such reproach. I have learned otherwise. I have learned that they're dangerous. I've also learned that I deserve better.

$$\diamond \ \diamond \ \diamond$$

March 1983

I reflected on how far I had come in the last thirteen years, and on how much further I wanted to go. Would I, I wondered, ever consider therapy again for assistance with the journey I still wanted to make? I recalled a conversation from not so long ago.

"My therapist was almost an hour late for my session," the caller was explaining to me. "He had no excuse and no apology for me. He was just—late. An hour late. I was really angry and I told him so. 'My time is valuable,' I said to him, 'and I wish you would treat it so.'

"Do you think I was right, Ellen? Don't you think my time should be treated as valuable? Don't you think I was entitled to be angry at him for showing up so late without an explanation?"

The caller was not a student of Objectivism. She had never met Dr. Leonard. She had begun her therapy years ago, shortly after I had begun my own, and at the time, she had barely been able to utter her opinion, much less words of anger.

"I don't think you were only right. I think you were fabulous!" I was thinking of how far she had come. "You wouldn't be silent if a friend kept you waiting for an hour. Why should you treat your therapist any differently?"

She was on the verge of tears. Her voice was shaking and anxiety was swallowing her up. "He said it was *my* problem and we spent the session working on it. He said we might have to work on it again because I'm having trouble seeing why his being so late is *my* problem. He was the one who was late. He's always late! But somehow it's my problem." She had begun her session feeling certain about who was at fault. Now she wasn't sure.

It's ironic, I thought, following this conversation. The fact is, a therapist—any therapist—who is anything short of well-intended and healthy, needs only one tool to pave the road to the abuse of his patient. It's not her background, her philosophy, or transference—though they all help. It's her self-doubt. This is the manifestation of neurosis that binds the most vulnerable patients to the most destructive therapists. This is the doctor's key to manipulating the patient into a role that serves only his purpose. Without it, his other weapons are ineffectual. But only if her self-esteem, confidence, and better judgment are securely locked in place, is she protected from the unethical psychotherapist. The irony? Such a person is unlikely to be seeking therapy.

Therapy? Again? Even with a non-Objectivist therapist? No, I thought. I don't think so. If I ever met a therapist who knew he was accountable for his actions, who didn't use his patients and confuse them to satisfy his own needs, who treated them fairly and with respect, who did not take advantage of their self-doubts, and who believed he should be constantly evaluated by those he treated, then maybe I would consider it. Maybe. But it's not likely to happen, I thought. Not likely at all.

EPILOGUE

As of the trial date, Lonnie Franklin Leonard was said to be living in Lake Gem, Florida, where he works as a beekeeper. In August of 1977, following the closing of his practice, Dr. Leonard surrendered his license to the State of New York, thereby avoiding an investigation and hearing by the state, as well as possible suspension of his license. The state erroneously accepted his license, terminating all action in the case. When their mistake was uncovered four years later, the file was returned to New York State for proper handling. In April of 1983, however, Ms. Chris Hyman of the State's Office of Professional Medical Conduct confirmed that no further action had been taken—nor would it be. Given that Dr. Leonard is presently living in Florida, "other cases are more compelling," she said. Dr. Leonard is still licensed to practice medicine and psychiatry.

Allan Blumenthal, M.D., is still practicing psychiatry in New York City.

Patricia Osborne, a nurse and nursing instructor, returned to her home in Maryland following the trial and resumed her work. She was said to be considering final pursuit of her educational goals, a Ph.D. in nursing. When asked at the trial's conclusion if she had any fear of retaliation from Dr. Leonard, Patti answered, "Whatever he might do to me now can't be any worse than what he's already done. Even if he killed me, he would just be putting me out of my pain." Today, she lives in North Carolina, where she teaches nursing and is pursuing that Ph.D. she wanted. She tells me she has finally found happiness. I believe her.

In late November 1982, the last remaining case against Dr. Leonard went to trial. That plaintiff's case had not been settled with Patti's and mine, as the dates of her treatment under Dr. Leonard placed liability with a different malpractice insurance carrier. The case of *Breitbard* vs. *Leonard* went to the jury, which awarded her $230,000. The judge reduced the award to $175,000.

Tony returned to Greg's and my life in the summer of 1982. He confirmed that, after four years of piecing his life back together again, I had, indeed, been *the baby in the bathwater*. His new understanding, coupled with his courage and honesty, made resumption of our relationship possible. Today, he is more than my brother-in-law. He is once again my close friend.

The mystery behind Linda's behavior remains unsolved, and the reasons behind her abandonment of her lawsuit against Dr. Leonard are still not known for sure. My attempts to contact Linda in an effort to reestablish a line of communication were, up until October of 1984, ignored. At that time, I telephoned her on a matter concerning the release of this book. During that brief conversation, she told me that she viewed my behavior toward her at the end of our relationship as "bizarre and neurotic." Further, she claimed that it was I who had stopped speaking to her. But my offer to discuss the events which Greg and I recalled so differently was coldly declined.

As of this writing, I have relocated with Greg, one more time, to the Northeast, where I am presently a second-year law student. Even my dreams survived.

I am more in love with Greg every day, as he continues to provide not only love and moral support, but joy, as well. He touches my life daily with his quick wit and boundless humor. He tolerates all my shortcomings with his endless patience, the same patience he showed during much more stressful times. But most importantly, he enriches my life with an intimate honesty and openness that has taught me how to trust again.

I have worked diligently at piecing together the fragments of my life that were my childhood, and at putting to rest the decade of my life that was spent on Dr. Leonard. This book, in large part, was as much the process as it was the product of that endeavor. It forced me back to times and places I would have preferred to avoid, but such travels back were necessary to find the answer to the question that had haunted me from the time of the trial's conclusion: How did it all happen? For until I understood that, I could never be certain that it would not happen again.

The rewards of the journey have been more than just the peace I was hoping would come from unlocking memories and retracing events. The rewards are greater than the security that comes from knowing that another Dr. Leonard could not happen to me again. Today, my life is full and rich. I am a strong, thriving, independent woman who knows where she's going, where she's been, and who she is. For the first time in my life, I feel whole.

Today, I am happier than I ever thought was possible.

It was twelve and a half years ago that I had my first session with Dr. Leonard. I had just turned twenty-one. The suit I filed against him five and a half years later was settled on November

5, 1982, only three days before my thirty-second birthday. In total, one third of my life, in one way or another, has been connected to Dr. Leonard. But before this period of my life could be brought to a satisfactory end, there was yet one need to be fulfilled.

I had filed my suit against Lonnie Franklin Leonard, M.D., with two goals in mind: to reassert my control in a relationship previously dictated by my former therapist, and to effect a permanent record of what he was and what he had done to me. The filing of my own suit, as well as the culmination of Patti's, left me content with the results of the first objective, but the premature conclusion to those cases left my second goal unattained.

This book is the making of that permanent record. This is my achievement of that second goal. This is my testimony.